CHOOSING HEALTH HIGH SCHOOL

MW01042242

BODY IMAGE AND EATING DISORDERS

Susan C. Giarratano, EdD, CHES

ETR Associates
Santa Cruz, California
1997

ETR Associates (Education, Training and Research) is a nonprofit organization committed to fostering the health, well-being and cultural diversity of individuals, families, schools and communities. The publishing program of ETR Associates provides books and materials that empower young people and adults with the skills to make positive health choices. We invite health professionals to learn more about our high-quality publishing, training and research programs by contacting us at P.O. Box 1830, Santa Cruz, CA 95061-1830, (800) 321-4407.

Susan Giarratano, EdD, CHES, is a professor in the health education program of the Health Sciences Department at California State University, Long Beach, where she coordinates the school health and teacher preparation program. She was codirector for 2 grants funded by the U.S. Department of Education to investigate the effects of a collaborative effort of health education, physical education, school nursing and child nutrition within a comprehensive school health education program. Currently, she is serving a term in an intergovernmental personnel agreement with the Centers for Disease Control and Prevention, Division of Adolescent and School Health. She has been a consultant for health education and minority health for public television, and has taught at the secondary school level. She is the author of *Choosing Health High School: Tobacco, Alcohol and Drugs*; an elementary health series; and a health education theory and application text.

Choosing Health High School
  Abstinence
  Body Image and Eating Disorders
  Communication and Self-Esteem
  Fitness and Health
  STD and HIV
  Sexuality and Relationships
  Tobacco, Alcohol and Drugs
  Violence and Injury

Series Editor: Kathleen Middleton, MS, CHES
Text design: Graphic Elements
Illustrations: Paul Tokmakian, Ann Smiley

© 1997 ETR Associates
All rights reserved. Published by ETR Associates,
P.O. Box 1830, Santa Cruz, CA 95061-1830

Reproduction permission is granted for masters
used within a single classroom only. Masters are
listed in the Table of Contents. Reproduction for
an entire school or school district is unlawful and
strictly prohibited.

Printed in the United States of America

10 9 8 7 6 5 4 3 2 1
ISBN 1-56071-519-7

Title No. H681

CONTENTS

Program Overview

The Body Image and Eating Disorders Resource Book

Anatomy of a Unit

Contents

CONTENTS

Appendixes

Masters

Unit 1 **1.1** What's Perfect?

1.2 Looking at Myself

1.3 Survival Notes

1.4 Changes

Unit 2 **2.1** Body Image Pressures

2.2 Cultural Connections

2.3 Media Messages

Unit 3 **3.1** Check Your Knowledge

3.2 What Causes Eating Disorders?

3.3 What Is Anorexia Nervosa?

3.4 What Is Bulimia?

3.5 Drugs and Eating Disorders

Unit 4 **4.1** Privacy Circles

4.2 Prevention Pointers

4.3 Help for Eating Disorders

4.4 Problems Eating You?

Final Evaluation

Jeopardy Game Board

ACKNOWLEDGMENTS

Choosing Health High School was made possible with the assistance of dedicated curriculum developers, teachers and health professionals. This program evolved from *Entering Adulthood*, the high school component of the *Contemporary Health Series*. The richness of this new program is demonstrated by the pool of talented professionals involved in both the original and the new versions.

Developers

Nancy Abbey
ETR Associates
Santa Cruz, California

Clint E. Bruess, EdD, CHES
University of Alabama at Birmingham
Birmingham, Alabama

Dale W. Evans, HSD, CHES
California State University, Long Beach
Long Beach, California

Susan C. Giarratano, EdD, CHES
California State University, Long Beach
Long Beach, California

Betty M. Hubbard, EdD, CHES
University of Central Arkansas
Conway, Arkansas

Lisa K. Hunter, PhD
Health & Education Communication Consultants
Berkeley, California

Susan J. Laing, MS, CHES
Department of Veterans Affairs Medical Center
Birmingham, Alabama

Donna Lloyd-Kolkin, PhD
Health & Education Communication Consultants
New Hope, Pennsylvania

Jeanie M. White, EdM, CHES
Education Consultant
Keizer, Oregon

Reviewers and Consultants

Brian Adams
Family Planning Council of Western Massachusetts
Northampton, Massachusetts

Janel Siebern Bartlett, MS, CHES
Dutchess County BOCES
Poughkeepsie, NY

Lori J. Bechtel, PhD
Pennsylvania State University, Altoona Campus
Altoona, Pennsylvania

Judith M. Boswell, RN, MS, CHES
University of New Mexico
Albuquerque, New Mexico

Marika Botha, PhD
Lewis and Clark State College
Lewiston, Idaho

Wanda Bunting
Newark Unified School District
Newark, California

John Daniels
Golden Sierra High School
Garden Valley, California

Joyce V. Fetro, PhD, CHES
San Francisco Unified School District
San Francisco, California

Mark L. Giese, EdD, FACSM
Northeastern State University
Tahlequah, Oklahoma

Karen Hart, MS, CHES
San Francisco Unified School District
San Francisco, California

Janet L. Henke
Old Court Middle School
Randallstown, Maryland

Russell G. Henke, MEd
Montgomery County Public Schools
Rockville, Maryland

Jon W. Hisgen, MS
Pewaukee Public Schools
Waukesha, Wisconsin

Bob Kampa
Gilroy High School
Gilroy, California

Freya Klein Kaufmann, MS, CHES
New York Academy of Medicine
New York, New York

David M. Macrina, PhD
University of Alabama at Birmingham
Birmingham, Alabama

Linda D. McDaniel, MS
Van Buren Middle School
Van Buren, Arkansas

Robert McDermott, PhD
University of South Florida
Tampa, Florida

ACKNOWLEDGMENTS

Carole McPherson, MA
Mentor Teacher Mission Hill Junior High School
Santa Cruz, California

Robert Mischell, MD
University of California, Berkeley
Berkeley, California

Donna Muto, MS
Mount Ararat School
Topsham, Maine

Priscilla Naworski, MS, CHES
California Department of Education
Healthy Kids Resource Center
Alameda County Office of Education
Alameda, California

Norma Riccobuono
La Paloma High School
Brentwood, California

Mary Rose-Colley, DEd, CHES
Lock Haven University
Lock Haven, Pennsylvania

Judith K. Scheer, MEd, EdS, CHES
Contra Costa County Office of Education
Walnut Creek, California

Michael A. Smith, MS, CHES
Long Beach Unified School District
Long Beach, California

Janet L. Sola, PhD
YWCA of the U.S.A.
New York, New York

Susan K. Telljohnn, HSD
University of Toledo
Toledo, Ohio

Donna J. Underwood, MS
Consulting Public Health Administrator
Champaign, Illinois

Peggy Woosley
Stuttgart Public Schools
Stuttgart, Arkansas

Dale Zevin, MA
Educational Consultant
Watsonville, California

COMPONENTS

PROGRAM GOAL

Students will acquire the necessary skills and information to make healthy choices.

Choosing Health High School consists of 8 Teacher/Student Resource books in critical topics appropriate for the high school health curriculum. *Think, Choose, Act Healthy, High School* provides creative activities to augment the basic program. There are also 13 *Health Facts* books that provide additional content information for teachers.

- **Teacher/Student Resource Books**—These 8 books address key health topics, content and issues for high school students. All teacher/student information, instructional process, assessment tools and student activity masters for the particular topic are included in each book.

- *Think, Choose, Act Healthy, High School*—This book provides 150 reproducible student activities that work hand in hand with the teacher/student resource books. They will challenge students to think and make their own personal health choices.

- *Health Facts* **Books**—These reference books provide clear, concise background information to support the resource books.

PROGRAM OVERVIEW

COMPONENTS

Health Facts Books Correlation	
Resource Books	***Health Facts* Books**
Abstinence	Abstinence Sexuality
Body Image and Eating Disorders	Nutrition and Body Image
Communication and Self-Esteem	Self-Esteem and Mental Health
Fitness and Health	Fitness
STD and HIV	STD HIV Disease
Sexuality and Relationships	Sexuality
Tobacco, Alcohol and Drugs	Drugs Tobacco
Violence and Injury	Violence Injury Prevention

PROGRAM OVERVIEW

TEACHING STRATEGIES

Each resource book is designed so you can easily find the instructional content, process and skills. You can spend more time on teaching and less on planning. Special tools are provided to help you challenge your students, reach out to their families and assess student success.

A wide variety of learning opportunities is provided in each book to increase interest and meet the needs of different kinds of learners. Many are interactive, encouraging students to help each other learn. The **31** teaching strategies can be divided into 4 categories based on educational purpose. They are Informational, Creative Expression, Sharing Ideas and Opinions and Developing Critical Thinking. Descriptions of the teaching strategies are found in the appendix.

Providing Key Information

Students need information before they can move to higher-level thinking. This program uses a variety of strategies to provide the information students need to take actions for health. Strategies include:

- anonymous question box
- current events
- demonstrations
- experiments
- games and puzzles

- guest speakers
- information gathering
- interviewing
- oral presentations

Encouraging Creative Expression

Creative expression provides the opportunity to integrate language arts, fine arts and personal experience into learning. It also allows students the opportunity to demonstrate their understanding in ways that are unique to them. Creative expression encourages students to capitalize on their strengths and their interests. Strategies include:

- artistic expression
- creative writing

- dramatic presentations
- roleplays

TEACHING STRATEGIES

Sharing Ideas, Feelings and Opinions

In the sensitive area of health education, providing a safe atmosphere in which to discuss a variety of opinions and feelings is essential. Discussion provides the opportunity to clarify misinformation and correct misconceptions. Strategies include:

- brainstorming
- class discussion
- clustering
- continuum voting
- dyad discussion
- family discussion
- forced field analysis
- journal writing
- panel discussion
- self-assessment
- small groups
- surveys and inventories

Developing Critical Thinking

Critical thinking skills are crucial if students are to adopt healthy behaviors. Healthy choices necessitate the ability to become independent thinkers, analyze problems and devise solutions in real-life situations. Strategies include:

- case studies
- cooperative learning groups
- debates
- factual writing
- media analysis
- personal contracts
- research

PROGRAM OVERVIEW

SKILLS INFUSION

Studies of high-risk children and adolescents show that certain characteristics are common to children who succeed in adverse situations. These children are called resilient. Evaluation of educational programs designed to build resiliency has shown that several elements are important for success. The most important is the inclusion of activities designed to build personal and social skills.

Throughout each resource book, students practice skills along with the content addressed in the activities. Activities that naturally infuse personal and social skills are identified.

- **Communication**—Students with effective communication skills are able to express thoughts and feelings, actively listen to others, and give clear verbal and nonverbal messages related to health or any other aspect of their lives.

- **Decision Making**—Students with effective decision-making skills are able to identify decision points, gather information, and analyze and evaluate alternatives before they take action. This skill is important to promote positive health choices.

- **Assertiveness**—Students with effective assertiveness skills are able to resist pressure and influence from peers, advertising or others that may be in conflict with healthy behavior. This skill involves the ability to negotiate in stressful situations and refuse unwanted influences.

- **Stress Management**—Students with effective stress-management skills are able to cope with stress as a normal part of life. They are able to identify situations and conditions that produce stress and adopt healthy coping behaviors.

- **Goal Setting**—Students with effective goal-setting skills are able to clarify goals based on their needs and interests. They are able to set realistic goals, identify the sub-steps to goals, take action and evaluate their progress. They are able to learn from mistakes and change goals as needed.

WORKING WITH FAMILIES AND COMMUNITIES

A few general principles can help you be most effective in teaching about health:

- Establish a rapport with your students, their families and your community.
- Prepare yourself so that you are comfortable with the content and instructional process required to teach about fitness and health successfully.
- Be aware of state laws and guidelines established by your school district that relate to health.
- Invite parents and other family members to attend a preview of the materials.

Family involvement improves student learning. Encourage family members and other volunteers to help you in the classroom as you teach these activities.

The Body Image and Eating Disorders Resource book

Why Teach About Body Image and Eating Disorders?

American culture is obsessed with appearance. Slenderness is a major preoccupation in our society. This focus on a single physical "ideal" for both men and women has produced a population overly concerned with body weight, as well as a multimillion-dollar diet industry.

The media contributes to our national fascination with thinness by a constant barrage of advertisements and programs that feature slender, well-proportioned females and lean, athletic males with well-defined muscles as models. Overweight people are usually depicted in the media for humorous purposes or weight control promotions. The people who are shown as living desirable, rewarding lives are slender and good looking. These messages affect perceptions of body image for everyone—adults, children and adolescents.

Body Image, Eating Disorders and High School Students

Most adolescents are preoccupied with the growth and physical changes in their bodies. This is quite normal. During adolescence they are also developing mental and emotional coping mechanisms to deal with those changes. However, the national obsession with thinness puts additional pressure on young people, whose body images are in flux already as they adjust to the changes of puberty.

The problem is extensive. Children as young as 5 years old have been found to be preoccupied with dieting because they fear being fat. A recent study examined attitudes among third through sixth graders from middle-income neighborhoods. It found that a large percentage of 8- to 13-year-old boys and girls wanted to be thinner and said they had already tried to lose weight.

Some dieting behaviors among adolescents may be considered within the range of normal. But obsession with the pursuit of thinness and weight control may be a severe psychological problem that needs competent professional assistance. Most eating disorders begin in the teen years. It is estimated that 10–15% of adolescent girls are affected by eating disorders. Although the figures are lower for males, it is clear that boys, too, feel pressures around body image.

This resource book focuses on issues related to body image, self-esteem, eating disorders and normal eating habits for adolescents. The learning activities enable students to identify positive attitudes and perceptions about body image, both from an individual and peer perspective, with an eye to developing a more accurate

(continued...)

THE BODY IMAGE AND EATING DISORDERS RESOURCE BOOK

WHY TEACH ABOUT BODY IMAGE AND EATING DISORDERS?

assessment of personal body image. The activities include an overview of anorexia nervosa and bulimia, the eating disorders most likely to affect teens. Indicators of each disorder, treatment and resources for help are discussed. Students are also encouraged to seek adult help if they or someone they know show signs of an eating disorder.

Background Information About Body Image and Eating Disorders

Instant Expert sections throughout this book give you all the information you need to teach each unit.

THE BODY IMAGE AND EATING DISORDERS RESOURCE BOOK

OBJECTIVES

Students Will Be Able to:

Unit 1: Body Image and Self-Esteem

1. Define body image and self-esteem.
2. Assess personal body image perception.
3. Identify realistic ways to improve body image.

Unit 2: Pressures on Body Image

1. Identify influences on body image.
3. Evaluate body image messages in advertising.

Unit 3: Eating Disorders

1. Identify the characteristics of eating disorders.
2. Explain the relationship between eating disorders and body image.

Unit 4: Help for Eating Disorders

1. Illustrate prevention behaviors for eating disorders.
2. Differentiate between normal teenage eating behaviors and eating disorder behaviors.

ANATOMY OF A UNIT

PREPARING TO TEACH

Objective identifies what students are expected to be able to do after instruction.

Getting Started lists preparation needed, including which masters to use.

Purpose states the rationale for the unit. **Main Points** are the key issues addressed. **Review** identifies the readings to increase your expertise in the content.

Vocabulary provides definitions of words used in the unit.

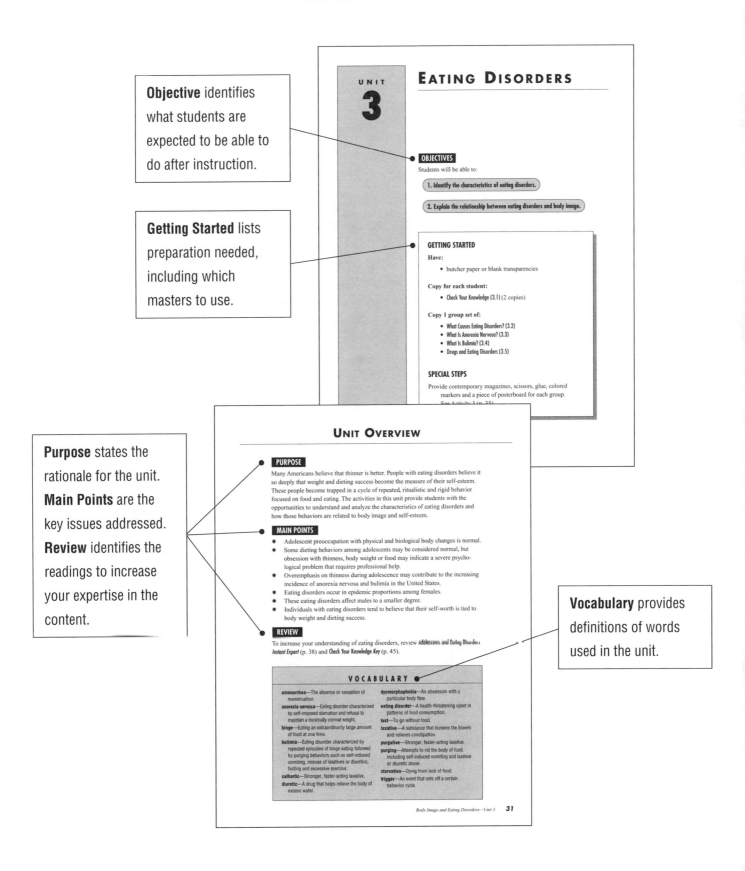

UNIT 3 — EATING DISORDERS

OBJECTIVES

Students will be able to:

1. Identify the characteristics of eating disorders.

2. Explain the relationship between eating disorders and body image.

GETTING STARTED

Have:

- butcher paper or blank transparencies

Copy for each student:

- Check Your Knowledge (3.1) (2 copies)

Copy 1 group set of:

- What Causes Eating Disorders? (3.2)
- What Is Anorexia Nervosa? (3.3)
- What Is Bulimia? (3.4)
- Drugs and Eating Disorders (3.5)

SPECIAL STEPS

Provide contemporary magazines, scissors, glue, colored markers and a piece of posterboard for each group. See Activity 3 (p. 35).

UNIT OVERVIEW

PURPOSE

Many Americans believe that thinner is better. People with eating disorders believe it so deeply that weight and dieting success become the measure of their self-esteem. These people become trapped in a cycle of repeated, ritualistic and rigid behavior focused on food and eating. The activities in this unit provide students with the opportunities to understand and analyze the characteristics of eating disorders and how those behaviors are related to body image and self-esteem.

MAIN POINTS

* Adolescent preoccupation with physical and biological body changes is normal.
* Some dieting behaviors among adolescents may be considered normal, but obsession with thinness, body weight or food may indicate a severe psychological problem that requires professional help.
* Overemphasis on thinness during adolescence may contribute to the increasing incidence of anorexia nervosa and bulimia in the United States.
* Eating disorders occur in epidemic proportions among females.
* These eating disorders affect males to a smaller degree.
* Individuals with eating disorders tend to believe that their self-worth is tied to body weight and dieting success.

REVIEW

To increase your understanding of eating disorders, review *Adolescents and Eating Disorders Instant Expert* (p. 38) and *Check Your Knowledge Key* (p. 45).

VOCABULARY

amenorrhea—The absence or cessation of menstruation.

anorexia nervosa—Eating disorder characterized by self-imposed starvation and refusal to maintain a minimally normal weight.

binge—Eating an extraordinarily large amount of food at one time.

bulimia—Eating disorder characterized by repeated episodes of binge eating followed by purging behaviors such as self-induced vomiting, misuse of laxatives or diuretics, fasting and excessive exercise.

cathartic—Stronger, faster-acting laxative.

diuretic—A drug that helps relieve the body of excess water.

dysmorphophobia—An obsession with a particular body flaw.

eating disorder—A health-threatening upset in patterns of food consumption.

fast—To go without food.

laxative—A substance that loosens the bowels and relieves constipation.

purgative—Stronger, faster-acting laxative.

purging—Attempts to rid the body of food, including self-induced vomiting and laxative or diuretic abuse.

starvation—Dying from lack of food.

trigger—An event that sets off a certain behavior cycle.

Body Image and Eating Disorders—Unit 3 **31**

ANATOMY OF A UNIT

TEACHING THE ACTIVITIES

Instant Expert pages provide concise background information for you. They follow each unit.

Process Cue identifies the teaching strategy used for the activity. Descriptions are in the Teaching Strategies appendix.

Building Skills icons identify activities that provide skill-specific practice.

Sharpen the Skill suggests ideas for more skills practice.

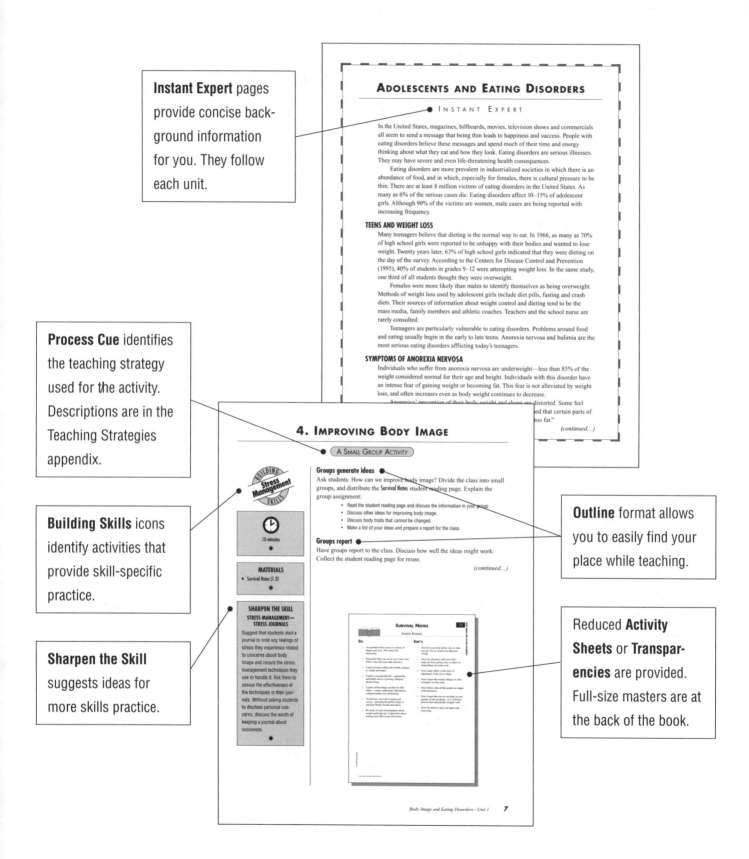

ADOLESCENTS AND EATING DISORDERS

INSTANT EXPERT

In the United States, magazines, billboards, movies, television shows and commercials all seem to send a message that being thin leads to happiness and success. People with eating disorders believe these messages and spend much of their time and energy thinking about what they eat and how they look. Eating disorders are serious illnesses. They may have severe and even life-threatening health consequences.

Eating disorders are more prevalent in industrialized societies in which there is an abundance of food, and in which, especially for females, there is cultural pressure to be thin. There are at least 8 million victims of eating disorders in the United States. As many as 6% of the serious cases die. Eating disorders affect 10–15% of adolescent girls. Although 90% of the victims are women, male cases are being reported with increasing frequency.

TEENS AND WEIGHT LOSS

Many teenagers believe that dieting is the normal way to eat. In 1966, as many as 70% of high school girls were reported to be unhappy with their bodies and wanted to lose weight. Twenty years later, 63% of high school girls indicated that they were dieting on the day of the survey. According to the Centers for Disease Control and Prevention (1995), 40% of students in grades 9–12 were attempting weight loss. In the same study, one third of all students thought they were overweight.

Females were more likely than males to identify themselves as being overweight. Methods of weight loss used by adolescent girls include diet pills, fasting and crash diets. Their sources of information about weight control and dieting tend to be the mass media, family members and athletic coaches. Teachers and the school nurse are rarely consulted.

Teenagers are particularly vulnerable to eating disorders. Problems around food and eating usually begin in the early to late teens. Anorexia nervosa and bulimia are the most serious eating disorders afflicting today's teenagers.

SYMPTOMS OF ANOREXIA NERVOSA

Individuals who suffer from anorexia nervosa are underweight—less than 85% of the weight considered normal for their age and height. Individuals with this disorder have an intense fear of gaining weight or becoming fat. This fear is not alleviated by weight loss, and often increases even as body weight continues to decrease.

Anorexics' perception of their body weight and shape are distorted. Some feel [...] that certain parts of [...] too fat."

(continued...)

4. IMPROVING BODY IMAGE

(A SMALL GROUP ACTIVITY)

Groups generate ideas

Ask students: How can we improve body image? Divide the class into small groups, and distribute the **Survival Notes** student reading page. Explain the group assignment:

- Read the student reading page and discuss the information in your group.
- Discuss other ideas for improving body image.
- Discuss body traits that *cannot* be changed.
- Make a list of your ideas and prepare a report for the class.

Groups report

Have groups report to the class. Discuss how well the ideas might work. Collect the student reading page for reuse.

(continued...)

BUILDING Stress Management SKILLS

🕐 10 minutes ✴

MATERIALS
- Survival Notes (1.3) ✴

SHARPEN THE SKILL
STRESS MANAGEMENT— STRESS JOURNALS
Suggest that students start a journal to note any feelings of stress they experience related to concerns about body image and record the stress management techniques they use to handle it. Ask them to assess the effectiveness of the techniques in their journals. Without asking students to disclose personal concerns, discuss the worth of keeping a journal about successes. ✴

SURVIVAL NOTES
STUDENT READING

DO:

DON'T:

Outline format allows you to easily find your place while teaching.

Reduced **Activity Sheets** or **Transparencies** are provided. Full-size masters are at the back of the book.

ANATOMY OF A UNIT

SPECIAL FEATURES

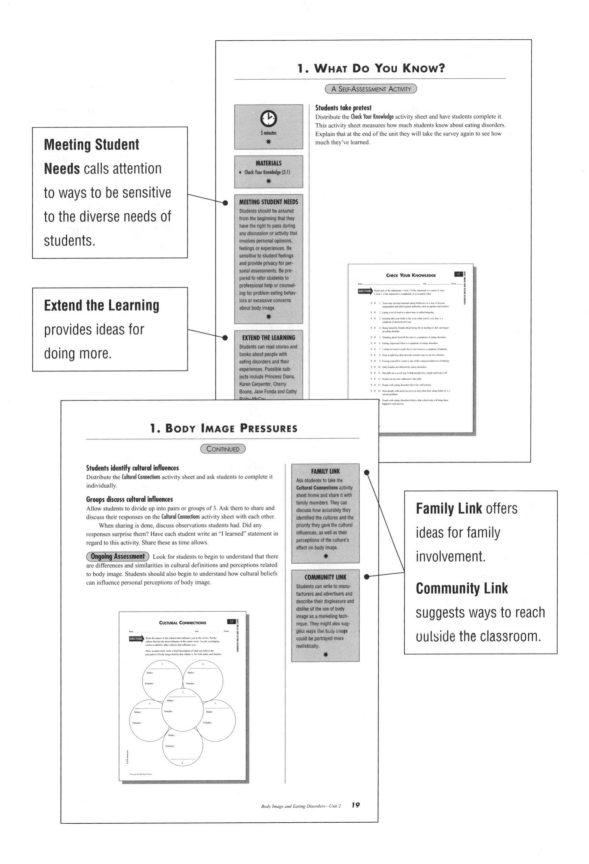

Meeting Student Needs calls attention to ways to be sensitive to the diverse needs of students.

Extend the Learning provides ideas for doing more.

Family Link offers ideas for family involvement.

Community Link suggests ways to reach outside the classroom.

1. WHAT DO YOU KNOW?

(A SELF-ASSESSMENT ACTIVITY)

Students take pretest
Distribute the **Check Your Knowledge** activity sheet and have students complete it. This activity sheet measures how much students know about eating disorders. Explain that at the end of the unit they will take the survey again to see how much they've learned.

5 minutes

MATERIALS
♦ Check Your Knowledge (3.1)

MEETING STUDENT NEEDS
Students should be assured from the beginning that they have the right to pass during any discussion or activity that involves personal opinions, feelings or experiences. Be sensitive to student feelings and provide privacy for personal assessments. Be prepared to refer students to professional help or counseling for problem eating behaviors or excessive concerns about body image.

EXTEND THE LEARNING
Students can read stories and books about people with eating disorders and their experiences. Possible subjects include Princess Diana, Karen Carpenter, Cherry Boone, Jane Fonda and Cathy Rigby-McCoy.

1. BODY IMAGE PRESSURES

(CONTINUED)

Students identify cultural influences
Distribute the **Cultural Connections** activity sheet and ask students to complete it individually.

Groups discuss cultural influences
Allow students to divide up into pairs or groups of 3. Ask them to share and discuss their responses on the **Cultural Connections** activity sheet with each other.
When sharing is done, discuss observations students had. Did any responses surprise them? Have each student write an "I learned" statement in regard to this activity. Share these as time allows.

(Ongoing Assessment) Look for students to begin to understand that there are differences and similarities in cultural definitions and perceptions related to body image. Students should also begin to understand how cultural beliefs can influence personal perceptions of body image.

FAMILY LINK
Ask students to take the **Cultural Connections** activity sheet home and share it with family members. They can discuss how accurately they identified the cultures and the priority they gave the cultural influences, as well as their perceptions of the culture's effect on body image.

COMMUNITY LINK
Students can write to manufacturers and advertisers and describe their displeasure and dislike of the use of body image as a marketing technique. They might also suggest ways that body image could be portrayed more realistically.

ANATOMY OF A UNIT

EVALUATION FEATURES

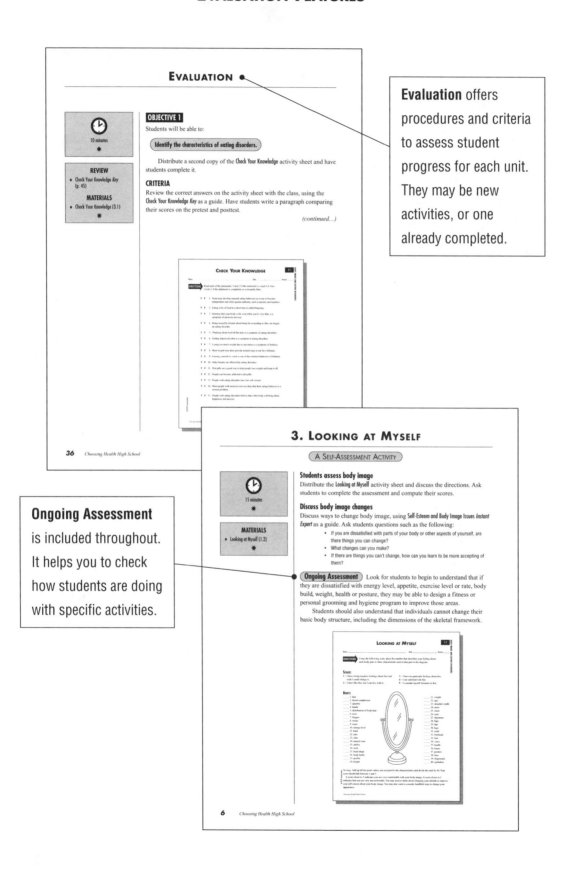

Evaluation offers procedures and criteria to assess student progress for each unit. They may be new activities, or one already completed.

Ongoing Assessment is included throughout. It helps you to check how students are doing with specific activities.

BODY IMAGE AND SELF-ESTEEM

TIME

2 periods

ACTIVITIES

1. What Is Perfection?

2. Defining Terms

3. Looking at Myself

4. Improving Body Image

BODY IMAGE AND SELF-ESTEEM

OBJECTIVES

Students will be able to:

> **1. Define body image and self-esteem.**

> **2. Assess personal body image perception.**

> **3. Identify realistic ways to improve body image.**

GETTING STARTED

Copy for each student:

- What's Perfect? (1.1)
- Looking at Myself (1.2)
- Changes (1.4)

Make classroom set of:

- Survival Notes (1.3)

UNIT OVERVIEW

PURPOSE

This unit helps students become aware of and understand the role that self-esteem and a positive body image play in achieving personal health.

MAIN POINTS

✳ Body image and self-esteem are related both to how you see yourself and to how others see you.

✳ Everyone has positive and negative points.

✳ Some body image characteristics can be changed and others cannot.

REVIEW

To increase your understanding of body image and self-esteem issues, review
Self-Esteem and Body Image Issues *Instant Expert* (p. 11).

VOCABULARY

body image—The way an individual views and believes others view his or her body.

ideal—An image or model thought of as perfect.

influence—The ability of a person or thing to affect others.

mental/emotional traits—Characteristics that relate to feelings, perceptions and relationships.

mental health—Psychological well-being; the capacity to cope with life situations.

perfect—Without flaw.

personal characteristics—Traits of an individual, including physical, mental/ emotional, social and personality traits.

personality traits—Attitudes, habits, emotions and thoughts that produce a characteristic way of behaving.

physical traits—Characteristics that relate to the body.

self-concept—A conscious set of beliefs about oneself that influence behavior.

self-esteem—Measure of how much a person values himself or herself.

social traits—Characteristics that provide the individual with a sense of self and others.

1. WHAT IS PERFECTION?

A CLASS DISCUSSION ACTIVITY

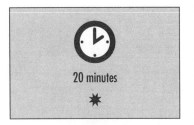

20 minutes

✷

MATERIALS

◆ What's Perfect? (1.1)

✷

MEETING STUDENT NEEDS

Body image is a very personal topic. Students need to be sensitive to the feelings of others during the lessons. You may want to set up or review class groundrules before teaching these units.

✷

Students describe perfect bodies

Distribute the What's Perfect? activity sheet and explain the directions. Ask students to complete Part 1—a description of the perfect body from the point of view of their own gender. They will not be sharing this description with others; it is for their own personal use.

Discuss influences on body image

When students have completed the description, discuss the things that influence how we define a *perfect* body? Responses may include:

- media—television, movies, videos, magazines, newspapers
- friends and peer groups
- parents and other family members
- what we see in the mirror

Students identify influences

Have students complete Part 2 of the activity sheet. They can use information from the class discussion to help them identify the things that influence their attitudes about body image. Students can keep this work confidential.

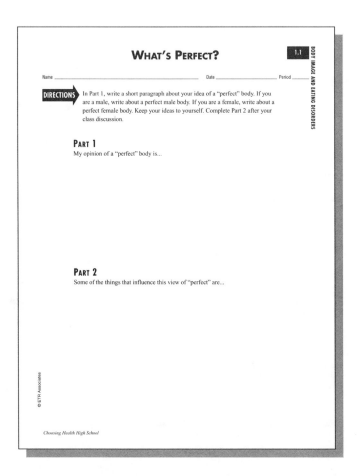

WHAT'S PERFECT?   1.1

Name _____ Date _____ Period _____

DIRECTIONS In Part 1, write a short paragraph about your idea of a "perfect" body. If you are a male, write about a perfect male body. If you are a female, write about a perfect female body. Keep your ideas to yourself. Complete Part 2 after your class discussion.

PART 1
My opinion of a "perfect" body is...

PART 2
Some of the things that influence this view of "perfect" are...

© ETR Associates

Choosing Health High School

2. DEFINING TERMS

Define self-esteem

Ask students to define *self-esteem.* Use the **Self-Esteem and Body Image Issues** *Instant Expert* to help students develop a definition.

Define body image

Ask students to define *body image.* Use the **Self-Esteem and Body Image Issues** *Instant Expert* to help students develop a definition.

Discuss terms

Discuss self-esteem and body image, using the **Self-Esteem and Body Image Issues** *Instant Expert* as a guide. Ask students: How are self-esteem and body image related to each other?

Ongoing Assessment Look for students to begin to understand that body image, or how well you like your body, and what you think of yourself are very important to self-esteem.

10 minutes

3. LOOKING AT MYSELF

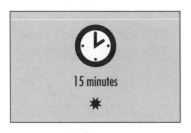

15 minutes

MATERIALS

♦ Looking at Myself (1.2)

Students assess body image

Distribute the Looking at Myself activity sheet and discuss the directions. Ask students to complete the assessment and compute their scores.

Discuss body image changes

Discuss ways to change body image, using Self-Esteem and Body Image Issues *Instant Expert* as a guide. Ask students questions such as the following:

* If you are dissatisfied with parts of your body or other aspects of yourself, are there things you can change?
* What changes can you make?
* If there are things you can't change, how can you learn to be more accepting of them?

Ongoing Assessment Look for students to begin to understand that if they are dissatisfied with energy level, appetite, exercise level or rate, body build, weight, health or posture, they may be able to design a fitness or personal grooming and hygiene program to improve those areas.

Students should also understand that individuals cannot change their basic body structure, including the dimensions of the skeletal framework.

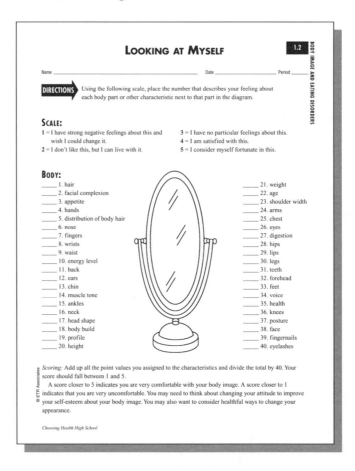

LOOKING AT MYSELF | 1.2 | BODY IMAGE AND EATING DISORDERS

Name _____ Date _____ Period _____

DIRECTIONS Using the following scale, place the number that describes your feeling about each body part or other characteristic next to that part in the diagram.

SCALE:

1 = I have strong negative feelings about this and wish I could change it.
2 = I don't like this, but I can live with it.

3 = I have no particular feelings about this.
4 = I am satisfied with this.
5 = I consider myself fortunate in this.

BODY:

____ 1. hair
____ 2. facial complexion
____ 3. appetite
____ 4. hands
____ 5. distribution of body hair
____ 6. nose
____ 7. fingers
____ 8. wrists
____ 9. waist
____ 10. energy level
____ 11. back
____ 12. ears
____ 13. chin
____ 14. muscle tone
____ 15. ankles
____ 16. neck
____ 17. head shape
____ 18. body build
____ 19. profile
____ 20. height

____ 21. weight
____ 22. age
____ 23. shoulder width
____ 24. arms
____ 25. chest
____ 26. eyes
____ 27. digestion
____ 28. hips
____ 29. lips
____ 30. legs
____ 31. teeth
____ 32. forehead
____ 33. feet
____ 34. voice
____ 35. health
____ 36. knees
____ 37. posture
____ 38. face
____ 39. fingernails
____ 40. eyelashes

Scoring: Add up all the point values you assigned to the characteristics and divide the total by 40. Your score should fall between 1 and 5.

A score closer to 5 indicates you are very comfortable with your body image. A score closer to 1 indicates that you are very uncomfortable. You may need to think about changing your attitude to improve your self-esteem about your body image. You may also want to consider healthful ways to change your appearance.

© ETR Associates

Choosing Health High School

4. IMPROVING BODY IMAGE

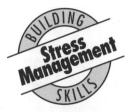

A SMALL GROUP ACTIVITY

Groups generate ideas

Ask students: How can we improve body image? Divide the class into small groups, and distribute the **Survival Notes** student reading page. Explain the group assignment:

- Read the student reading page and discuss the information in your group.
- Discuss other ideas for improving body image.
- Discuss body traits that *cannot* be changed.
- Make a list of your ideas and prepare a report for the class.

Groups report

Have groups report to the class. Discuss how well the ideas might work. Collect the student reading page for reuse.

(continued...)

10 minutes

✳

MATERIALS

◆ Survival Notes (1.3)

✳

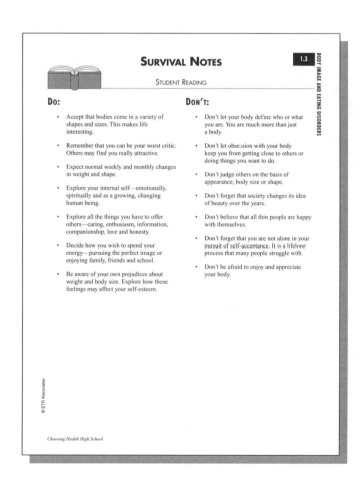

SURVIVAL NOTES | 1.3

STUDENT READING

DO:

- Accept that bodies come in a variety of shapes and sizes. This makes life interesting.

- Remember that you can be your worst critic. Others may find you really attractive.

- Expect normal weekly and monthly changes in weight and shape.

- Explore your internal self—emotionally, spiritually and as a growing, changing human being.

- Explore all the things you have to offer others—caring, enthusiasm, information, companionship, love and honesty.

- Decide how you wish to spend your energy—pursuing the perfect image or enjoying family, friends and school.

- Be aware of your own prejudices about weight and body size. Explore how those feelings may affect your self-esteem.

DON'T:

- Don't let your body define who or what you are. You are much more than just a body.

- Don't let obsession with your body keep you from getting close to others or doing things you want to do.

- Don't judge others on the basis of appearance, body size or shape.

- Don't forget that society changes its idea of beauty over the years.

- Don't believe that all thin people are happy with themselves.

- Don't forget that you are not alone in your pursuit of self-acceptance. It is a lifelong process that many people struggle with.

- Don't be afraid to enjoy and appreciate your body.

© ETR Associates

Choosing Health High School

4. IMPROVING BODY IMAGE

SHARPEN THE SKILL

**STRESS MANAGEMENT—
STRESS JOURNALS**

Suggest that students start a journal to note any feelings of stress they experience related to concerns about body image and record the stress management techniques they use to handle it. Ask them to assess the effectiveness of the techniques in their journals. Without asking students to disclose personal concerns, discuss the worth of keeping a journal about successes.

Ongoing Assessment Look for students' ability to suggest ways to enhance body image. Possible suggestions:

- Look in a mirror. Note your positive features and think about how they can be enhanced.
- Look closely at the features or body parts you consider least attractive and reevaluate them.
- Put up photographs of yourself that you like.
- The next time you go to extra effort to look good, say aloud to the mirror, "I look great today."
- Pamper yourself with a new haircut or new clothes.
- Ask friends and family members what they find physically attractive about you.
- Work on your physical potential with exercise and healthy eating.
- Talk with other people if you feel lonely or isolated.
- Keep a mental list of the positive ways you've grown and changed.

EVALUATION

OBJECTIVE 1

Students will be able to:

> **Define body image and self-esteem.**

Have students write a definition of body image and a definition of self-esteem.

CRITERIA

See the **Self-Esteem and Body Image Issues** *Instant Expert* for evaluation criteria.

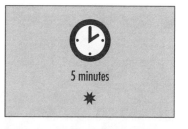

5 minutes

REVIEW

◆ Self-Esteem and Body Image Issues *Instant Expert* (p. 11)

OBJECTIVE 2

Students will be able to:

> **Assess personal body image perception.**

Ask students to review their responses on the **Looking at Myself** activity sheet. Ask them to describe 3 characteristics that they marked as 1s. They should discuss how each of the 3 characteristics influences or affects personal body image and/or self-esteem. Students may do this orally or in writing.

CRITERIA

See the **Self-Esteem and Body Image Issues** *Instant Expert* for evaluation criteria.

(continued...)

15 minutes

REVIEW

◆ Self-Esteem and Body Image Issues *Instant Expert* (p. 11)

MATERIALS

◆ completed Looking at Myself (1.2), from Activity 3

EVALUATION

10 minutes
✳

REVIEW

◆ Self-Esteem and Body Image Issues *Instant Expert* (p. 11)

MATERIALS

◆ Changes (1.4)

✳

OBJECTIVE 3

Students will be able to:

> Identify realistic ways to improve body image.

Distribute the **Changes** evaluation sheet and ask students to complete it. Ask students to choose realistic changes that could be accomplished within a few days or a week.

CRITERIA

Look for students understanding of steps to improve body image. See Ongoing Assessment for Activity 4 (p. 8) for evaluation criteria.

Students should also identify some aspect of their basic skeletal framework as something that cannot be changed.

CHANGES   1.4

BODY IMAGE AND EATING DISORDERS

Name _____ Date _____ Period _____

DIRECTIONS Look over your answers on the **Looking at Myself** activity sheet. Choose the body areas that you marked with a 1 or 2. List those areas in the columns below as something that can be changed or something that cannot be changed. After you make these lists, answer the questions.

THINGS I *CAN* CHANGE   **THINGS I *CANNOT* CHANGE**

_____   _____
_____   _____
_____   _____
_____   _____
_____   _____
_____   _____

1. Choose 1 of the things you *can* change: _____
Describe what change you *can* make: _____
How can you make this change?

2. Choose 1 of the things you *cannot* change: _____
How can you work at accepting this?

© ETR Associates

Choosing Health High School

SELF-ESTEEM AND BODY IMAGE ISSUES

Body image refers to the view people have of their physical selves. Developing a positive body image helps people see themselves as attractive, and is a prerequisite for developing a mature personal identity. Exploration, experimentation, communication and learning about oneself help a person develop a positive body image.

The way people feel about their physical selves affects their *self-esteem.* The California Task Force to Promote Self-Esteem and Personal and Social Responsibility defined self-esteem as "appreciating my own worth and importance and having the character to be accountable for myself and to act responsibly toward others." Self-esteem expresses an attitude of approval or disapproval of the self. It includes feelings of self-worth and the judgments people make about themselves, both positive and negative.

These judgments have an important effect on overall behavior. People with a positive body image usually have positive attitudes about other aspects of themselves. Personal level of wellness is affected by the ways people think about and value themselves. Those who like themselves and think about themselves in positive terms tend to be healthier.

INFLUENCES ON PHYSICAL APPEARANCE

Personal characteristics change during adolescence and early adulthood. These changes include the visible signs of puberty: growth spurts, development of reproductive organs and appearance of secondary sex characteristics. Adolescents also have a strong desire to look "normal," acceptable and pleasing to self and others.

Skin texture, complexion and teeth contribute in important ways to physical appearance. Clothing, grooming and personal hygiene (cleanliness, make-up, hairstyle) also have an effect. Three other factors also affect physical appearance:

- the dimensions (length and breadth) of the skeletal framework
- the distribution and development of the muscles resting upon the skeleton
- the amount and location of adipose tissue (fat) throughout the body

People's feelings about these factors contribute to their sense of body image. The first factor—the basic body framework—is a function of heredity and genetics and is essentially out of the individual's control. Individuals may be able to control or influence the other 2 factors, although heredity and genetics also play a role in the development of muscle mass and fat.

Although individuals cannot change their basic body structure, even people without the build of a fashion model, athlete or body builder can be fit.

(continued...)

SELF-ESTEEM AND BODY IMAGE ISSUES

IMPROVING BODY IMAGE AND SELF-ESTEEM

A realistic assessment of personal traits can be an important step in the development of high self-esteem and a good self-concept. Many people fail to recognize their positive qualities and focus only on their negative ones. In addition to physical characteristics, people possess mental/emotional, personality and social traits. These characteristics relate to a person's feelings, perceptions, attitudes, habits and behaviors both toward the self and others.

It helps to remember that everyone has some negative qualities. When people realistically consider *both* their positive and negative characteristics, they can decide to work on changing traits they consider negative. A sense of perspective is helpful. Awareness of one's good qualities, strengths and accomplishments can boost self-esteem and increase the chances of success in making changes in other qualities.

Having a positive self-concept and body image is *not* conceit. A realistic and healthful self-appraisal can be made without bragging or putting oneself down.

Adolescents are particularly vulnerable to body image concerns. The following steps can be useful to them in developing a positive body image.

Actions That Contribute to Positive Body Image

- Accept that bodies come in a variety of shapes and sizes. This makes life interesting.
- Remember that you can be your worst critic. Others may find you really attractive.
- Expect normal weekly and monthly changes in weight and shape.
- Explore your internal self—emotionally, spiritually and as a growing, changing human being.
- Explore all the things you have to offer others—caring, enthusiasm, information, companionship, love and honesty.
- Decide how you wish to spend your energy—pursuing the perfect image or enjoying family, friends and school.
- Be aware of your own prejudices about weight and body size. Explore how those feelings may affect your self-esteem.

(continued...)

SELF-ESTEEM AND BODY IMAGE ISSUES

Attitudes to Avoid

- Don't let your body define who or what you are. You are much more than just a body.
- Don't let obsession with your body keep you from getting close to others or doing things you want to do.
- Don't judge others on the basis of appearance, body size or shape.
- Don't forget that society changes its idea of beauty over the years.
- Don't believe that all thin people are happy with themselves.
- Don't forget that you are not alone in your pursuit of self-acceptance. It is a lifelong process that many people struggle with.
- Don't be afraid to enjoy and appreciate your body.

PRESSURES ON BODY IMAGE

TIME
2 periods

ACTIVITIES
1. Body Image Pressures
2. Messages from the Media

PRESSURES ON BODY IMAGE

OBJECTIVES

Students will be able to:

> 1. Identify influences on body image.

> 2. Evaluate body image messages in advertising.

GETTING STARTED

Copy for each student:

- Body Image Pressures (2.1)
- Cultural Connections (2.2)
- Media Messages (2.3) (2 copies)

SPECIAL STEPS

Ask students to cut out and bring to class at least 1 magazine or newspaper advertisement that they think contains messages about body image. See Activity 2 (p. 20).

UNIT OVERVIEW

PURPOSE

Social, cultural and historical beliefs about body image influence present-day perceptions about our physical selves. The mass media, family members and peers probably have the most influence on students. This unit helps students understand how culture and the media play important roles in influencing body image perception.

MAIN POINTS

✳ Shared knowledge, traditions, beliefs and values influence the thoughts and decisions people make about themselves as individuals and as a group.

✳ Cultural messages, including those from the media, family, society and peers influence the perception of body image.

✳ In American culture, print, broadcast and electronic media are powerful influences on the perceptions people have of themselves.

✳ Media literacy skills help us critically assess advertising messages and the perceptions of body image they evoke.

REVIEW

To increase your understanding of influences on body image, review **Culture and Body Image** *Instant Expert* (p. 24).

VOCABULARY

advertising—Public announcements of the qualities or advantages of a product or service.

body composition—The proportion of body muscle to body fat.

culture—Ideas, customs, skills and arts of a people or group.

electronic media—Media that require electricity to operate and communicate messages.

media—Means of communication that provide information and convey messages to the public.

media literacy—The ability to critically analyze and evaluate a variety of media.

obesity—A condition in which an excessive proportion of body tissue is fat; being 20% or more above desirable weight.

overweight—Being 10% or more above desirable weight.

1. BODY IMAGE PRESSURES

A CLASS DISCUSSION ACTIVITY

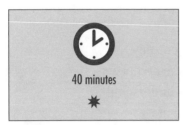

40 minutes

MATERIALS

♦ Body Image Pressures (2.1)
♦ Cultural Connections (2.2)

MEETING STUDENT NEEDS

Point out to students that they may have different perceptions about cultural beliefs and some of their beliefs may be based on stereotypes. Encourage them to be sensitive to cultural differences.

Students read about pressures

Distribute the **Body Image Pressures** student reading page. Have students read it individually, in small groups or aloud as a class.

Discuss pressures

Lead a class discussion of the pressures on both males and females to meet certain standards for physical appearance, using the **Culture and Body Image** *Instant Expert* as a guide. Ask students:

- What are some of the pressures males face around body image? What are some pressures females face?
- How are the pressures different for males and females?
- How are they alike?
- What are some of the differences in the ways males and females cope with these pressures?

Ask students to think about other ways our society and our culture pressure people to change or dislike their bodies. Note that *pressures* as well as *perceptions* around ideal body images can lead to eating disorders.

(continued...)

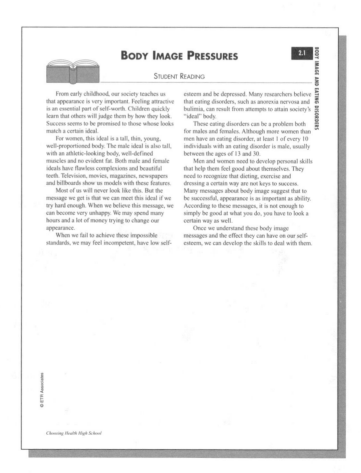

BODY IMAGE PRESSURES

2.1

STUDENT READING

From early childhood, our society teaches us that appearance is very important. Feeling attractive is an essential part of self-worth. Children quickly learn that others will judge them by how they look. Success seems to be promised to those whose looks match a certain ideal.

For women, this ideal is a tall, thin, young, well-proportioned body. The male ideal is also tall, with an athletic-looking body, well-defined muscles and no evident fat. Both male and female ideals have flawless complexions and beautiful teeth. Television, movies, magazines, newspapers and billboards show us models with these features.

Most of us will never look like this. But the message we get is that we can meet this ideal if we try hard enough. When we believe this message, we can become very unhappy. We may spend many hours and a lot of money trying to change our appearance.

When we fail to achieve these impossible standards, we may feel incompetent, have low self-

esteem and be depressed. Many researchers believe that eating disorders, such as anorexia nervosa and bulimia, can result from attempts to attain society's "ideal" body.

These eating disorders can be a problem both for males and females. Although more women than men have an eating disorder, at least 1 of every 10 individuals with an eating disorder is male, usually between the ages of 13 and 30.

Men and women need to develop personal skills that help them feel good about themselves. They need to recognize that dieting, exercise and dressing a certain way are not keys to success. Many messages about body image suggest that to be successful, appearance is as important as ability. According to these messages, it is not enough to simply be good at what you do, you have to look a certain way as well.

Once we understand these body image messages and the effect they can have on our self-esteem, we can develop the skills to deal with them.

© ETR Associates

Choosing Health High School

1. BODY IMAGE PRESSURES

CONTINUED

Students identify cultural influences

Distribute the Cultural Connections activity sheet and ask students to complete it individually.

Groups discuss cultural influences

Allow students to divide up into pairs or groups of 3. Ask them to share and discuss their responses on the Cultural Connections activity sheet with each other.

When sharing is done, discuss observations students had. Did any responses surprise them? Have each student write an "I learned" statement in regard to this activity. Share these as time allows.

Ongoing Assessment   Look for students to begin to understand that there are differences and similarities in cultural definitions and perceptions related to body image. Students should also begin to understand how cultural beliefs can influence personal perceptions of body image.

FAMILY LINK

Ask students to take the **Cultural Connections** activity sheet home and share it with family members. They can discuss how accurately they identified the cultures and the priority they gave the cultural influences, as well as their perceptions of the culture's effect on body image.

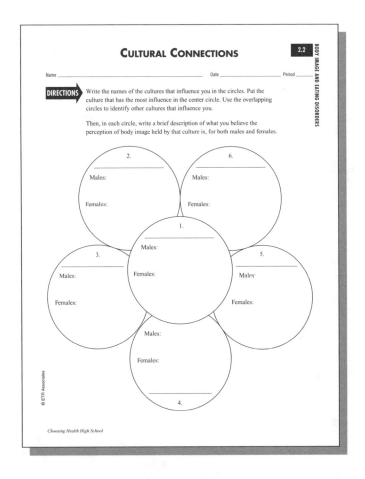

2. MESSAGES FROM THE MEDIA

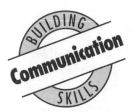

A MEDIA ANALYSIS ACTIVITY

25 minutes

❋

MATERIALS

- advertisements with body image messages
- Media Messages (2.3)

FAMILY LINK

Students can talk to a parent or other trusted adult about the body image criteria used by the media.

Discuss media influences

Ask students:

- How do the media influence perceptions and attitudes about body image?
- What role do television, movies and videos play in the development of body image?

Discuss billboard, magazine and newspaper advertisements that picture the use of drugs such as tobacco and alcohol as enjoyable. Ask students if these ads also influence body image.

Point out that many products (including cigarettes and alcoholic beverages) are used in ads that are targeted to a specific gender, culture or ethnic group. Ask students for examples of such advertisements.

(continued...)

MEDIA MESSAGES `2.3`

BODY IMAGE AND EATING DISORDERS

Name _____ Date _____ Period _____

DIRECTIONS Answer the questions about the advertisement you have. Use steps 1–4 in the *Scoring and Interpretation* section to analyze the results.

What is the name of the advertised product? _____

What kind of product is it? (Circle or fill in the blank.)

Diet (weight control)   Alcoholic beverage (beer, wine, liquor)
Clothing
Tobacco   Other _____

Rate the advertisement on each of the following factors, using this scale:

5 = Strongly Agree   **2** = Disagree
4 = Agree   **1** = Strongly Disagree
3 = Undecided   **0** = Not Applicable (no body-image messages included)

Circle 1 choice for each statement.

Generally, the advertisement: Score

1. Suggests that use of the product will produce a positive body image.   5 4 3 2 1 0 _____
2. Shows a socially negative body image.   5 4 3 2 1 0 _____
3. Suggests the product is a solution for boredom.   5 4 3 2 1 0 _____
4. Associates the use of the product with fun or pleasure.   5 4 3 2 1 0 _____
5. Associates the use of the product with being attractive.   5 4 3 2 1 0 _____
6. Encourages the use of the product as a method of problem-solving.   5 4 3 2 1 0 _____
7. Suggests that everyone is using the product.   5 4 3 2 1 0 _____
8. Suggests that people who use the product are mature.   5 4 3 2 1 0 _____
9. Shows a model using the product.   5 4 3 2 1 0 _____
10. Suggests that the product will improve performance   5 4 3 2 1 0 _____
    (intellectual, physical, spiritual, etc.).

Total Points _____

(continued...)

© ETR Associates

Choosing Health High School

---

2. MESSAGES FROM THE MEDIA

(CONTINUED)

Discuss physical characteristics

Ask students to describe some famous people's physical characteristics. You might want to list these on the board in separate columns for males and females. Ask students:

- How do these famous people's characteristics influence your view of your own body?
- If you have some similar features, how does this influence your personal perception of body image?
- If you have differences in your features, how does this influence your personal perception of body image?

Students analyze advertisements

Ask students to take out the advertisements they collected. Distribute the Media Messages activity sheet. Review the directions with students. Ask students to use the activity sheet to evaluate their advertisements.

Students report

Ask students to report on the messages they found in the advertisements. Ask each student:

- What were your final ratings from step 3 and step 4 of the activity sheet?
- How could the advertisement be changed to make it more accurate?

Ongoing Assessment Look for students to conclude that media messages seem to say that a slim and muscular body defines *attractive* for both men and women. They should understand that the media message is not a health message; it is not necessary to be slim and muscular to be healthy.

COMMUNITY LINK

Students can write to manufacturers and advertisers and describe their displeasure and dislike of the use of body image as a marketing technique. They might also suggest ways that body image could be portrayed more realistically.

EXTEND THE LEARNING

As a result of acquiring media literacy skills, students may become quite skeptical and cynical if the focus is placed only on the critical analysis of the messages. Encourage students to create their own versions of accurate and honest media messages.

EVALUATION

10 minutes

OBJECTIVE 1

Students will be able to:

> ### Identify influences on body image.

Divide the class into small groups. Ask groups to create lists of potential influences on body image. Ask them to include specific examples of each influence.

CRITERIA

Lists should include:

- media
- family and cultural perceptions
- specific physical characteristics
- self-esteem

(continued...)

EVALUATION

OBJECTIVE 2

Students will be able to:

> Evaluate body image messages in advertising.

Distribute a second copy of the **Media Messages** activity sheet. Have students use it to evaluate an advertisement on television. Ask students to complete the form, then comment in writing on how television differs from printed media.

CRITERIA

Look for students to conclude that print and television media messages have many similarities. The body defined as attractive often is slim and muscular.

20 minutes

REVIEW

◆ Culture and Body Image *Instant Expert* (p. 24)

MATERIALS

◆ Media Messages (2.3)

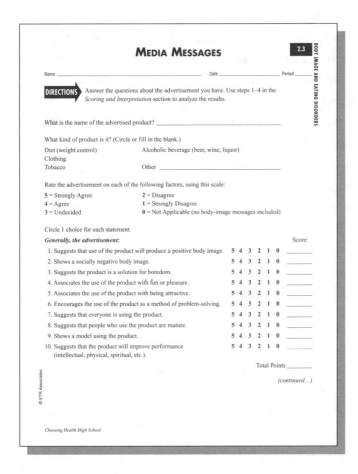

MEDIA MESSAGES `2.3`

BODY IMAGE AND EATING DISORDERS

Name _____ Date _____ Period _____

DIRECTIONS ➤ Answer the questions about the advertisement you have. Use steps 1–4 in the *Scoring and Interpretation* section to analyze the results.

What is the name of the advertised product? _____

What kind of product is it? (Circle or fill in the blank.)

Diet (weight control)   Alcoholic beverage (beer, wine, liquor)
Clothing
Tobacco   Other _____

Rate the advertisement on each of the following factors, using this scale:

5 = Strongly Agree   2 = Disagree
4 = Agree   1 = Strongly Disagree
3 = Undecided   0 = Not Applicable (no body-image messages included)

Circle 1 choice for each statement.

Generally, the advertisement: Score

1. Suggests that use of the product will produce a positive body image.   5 4 3 2 1 0 _____
2. Shows a socially negative body image.   5 4 3 2 1 0 _____
3. Suggests the product is a solution for boredom.   5 4 3 2 1 0 _____
4. Associates the use of the product with fun or pleasure.   5 4 3 2 1 0 _____
5. Associates the use of the product with being attractive.   5 4 3 2 1 0 _____
6. Encourages the use of the product as a method of problem-solving. 5 4 3 2 1 0 _____
7. Suggests that everyone is using the product.   5 4 3 2 1 0 _____
8. Suggests that people who use the product are mature.   5 4 3 2 1 0 _____
9. Shows a model using the product.   5 4 3 2 1 0 _____
10. Suggests that the product will improve performance   5 4 3 2 1 0 _____
    (intellectual, physical, spiritual, etc.).

Total Points _____

(continued...)

© ETR Associates

Choosing Health High School

CULTURE AND BODY IMAGE

Culture refers to the knowledge, traditions, beliefs and values that are developed, learned and shared by members of a society. These shared norms, beliefs and values influence individual thoughts and the decisions people make with regard to themselves, their families and others. Culture can be an important influence on body image.

However, while cultural norms are a useful concept for describing a group in general terms, there is much intracultural variation. People from the same culture may have very different diets, eating behaviors and perceptions of desirable body weight.

CULTURAL STANDARDS

Definitions of the ideal body size and shape vary from one culture to another. Slenderness has become a major preoccupation for many Americans, who consider a slim figure both attractive and healthy, and associate slimness with success.

In contrast, obesity is idealized in other cultures. Being overweight is seen as a sign of wealth, and the luxury of inactivity and overeating as a sign of good health. Polynesians, Samoans and past European societies have admired the obese.

Whatever its particular standard, culture shapes our perceptions of "ideal" body weight and shape. As early as age 5 or 6, children begin to acquire the cultural criteria used by adults for judging physical attractiveness. In several studies, children tended to condemn other children who were overweight or obese in a culture where slimness is valued and used pejorative terms to describe them.

Overweight people may face discrimination in educational and employment opportunities as well as personal relationships. Society's negative attitudes toward obesity may affect personal social and economic conditions, particularly for young women. One study found that overweight young women had completed fewer years of school, were less likely to marry, more likely to be poor and earned lower wages than normal weight women. Overweight men were not as likely to marry as normal weight men, but their earnings were not affected by being overweight.

It is extremely difficult for people to separate themselves from cultural standards. It is even more difficult to see that the body shapes we most admire reflect the taste of our times rather than an absolute aesthetic.

DEFINING "IDEAL" WEIGHT

Medically, ideal or desirable weight is usually determined by gender and in terms of height. But, because relative amounts of fat, lean (muscle) tissue and bone size vary greatly from person to person, ideal weights are given as ranges in recommended weight tables.

(continued...)

CULTURE AND BODY IMAGE

Some experts have challenged the recommended weight tables. They suggest that the concept of ideal weight should be more flexible; because health hazards are associated only with extreme overweight (obesity) and underweight—20% over or under ideal range—efforts to change body weight should focus on those people at the extremes, rather than on those whose weights deviate only minimally from the ideal.

It is also important to examine body composition to be sure that the percentage of weight over the average is contributed by an excess of body fat and not body muscle. (Muscle weighs 4 times more than fat.) A weight lifter might be "overweight"—heavier than average—but this excess weight is due to body muscle. Therefore, the weight lifter would not be considered obese.

THE AMERICAN "IDEAL"

Since the 1960s, American culture has placed an extraordinary emphasis on a slim female body. If fat is bad, then thin is good, thinner is better, and thinnest is best. The present American feminine ideal is thin and firm. The male image promoted as ideal is tall and athletic, with well-defined muscles.

In the 1980s, the typical Miss America was between 5'6" and 5'11" tall and weighed 110–120 pounds. She exercised an average of 14 hours per week and had small hips and large breasts—almost a physical impossibility for someone of that height and weight.

The aesthetic ideal has grown consistently leaner over time and is now much thinner than the health ideal. In recent years, Jane Fonda's slim, toned body type became the rage. However, magazines and journals later reported that she had an eating disorder, bulimia nervosa, that affected her for 20 years. Diana, Princess of Wales, and Cathy Rigby-McCoy of Olympic and exercise equipment fame have also gone public with their struggles with bulimia. Eighty percent of adult women, as reported in Vogue magazine in 1986, felt they were "too fat" and wanted to be thinner. Men too strive for unrealistic standards for body shape and size. (Wolf, 1991; Silverstein et al., 1986; Wiseman et al., 1992.)

(continued...)

CULTURE AND BODY IMAGE

Brownell and Wadden (1992) identify 2 assumptions underlying the search for the ideal body weight:

- The body can be shaped and molded at will. With the right diet, exercise program and personal effort, an individual can have the "perfect" weight and contours.
- The benefits justify the search. Having the ideal body will bring vast rewards (e.g., interpersonal attraction, professional development, wealth and happiness).

These beliefs have led to unprecedented levels of dieting, exercise and plastic surgery in the United States. The diet industry has become a multimillion-dollar business as people turn to diet pills, sodas, drinks and other potions in their quest for thinness. Weight-loss books are best sellers. Exercise spas and weight-loss clinics, clubs and enrollment programs are booming. Exercise equipment sales for at-home use are at an all-time high. However, the prevalence of obesity (defined as being 20% or more above desirable weight) has doubled since 1900. Despite our nation's preoccupation with dieting, people have actually grown heavier in recent years.

Many people are obsessed not only with weight, but with other perceived body imperfections. Movie stars and others submit to cosmetic surgery in an attempt to obtain a flawless appearance. Nose jobs, liposuction, tummy and buttock tucks, breast implants and rib removal are commonly used in the search for the perfect body.

THE MEDIA INFLUENCE

We receive hundreds and thousands of messages every day through a variety of media. Today's media include television (including music videos), radio, newspapers, billboards, magazines, advertising, on-line communication (the Internet and the World Wide Web), and the arts. The images people see in the various media often have a strong influence on body image.

Models, actors and other media figures most often are slim, with well-proportioned, well-defined figures. Overweight or heavier-than-average people are seldom featured, and often depicted as comical figures when they are.

Advertisements also use attractive, well-proportioned, slim models. They often show these men and women having fun together and imply that use of the featured product will attract others. The product is usually shown being used in an exciting or beautiful setting.

(continued...)

CULTURE AND BODY IMAGE

The fashion industry also plays a major role in dictating the "body ideal"—a body type that most women and men do not have. Fashion models are chosen for their height, broad shoulders, narrow hips and long legs. Over the last 30 years, the look of fashion models has changed to be even taller and thinner, with bust and hip size decreasing in relation to waist size.

MEDIA LITERACY

Media literacy is the ability to critically interpret the many messages put out by the media. It includes the skills used to assess and judge the accuracy and integrity of the information provided by the media. It also includes the ability to challenge, to question and to formulate opinions about the source of the message and its content.

Media literacy skills can be invaluable to students as they seek to establish a healthy body image in the midst of media and cultural messages that promote one set "ideal" and do not reflect the reality of body size diversity.

EATING DISORDERS

TIME

2 periods

ACTIVITIES

1. What Do You Know?
2. Learning About Eating Disorders
3. Influences on Eating Disorders

UNIT 3

EATING DISORDERS

OBJECTIVES

Students will be able to:

> 1. Identify the characteristics of eating disorders.

> 2. Explain the relationship between eating disorders and body image.

GETTING STARTED

Have:

- butcher paper or blank transparencies

Copy for each student:

- Check Your Knowledge (3.1) (2 copies)

Copy 1 group set of:

- What Causes Eating Disorders? (3.2)
- What Is Anorexia Nervosa? (3.3)
- What Is Bulimia? (3.4)
- Drugs and Eating Disorders (3.5)

SPECIAL STEPS

Provide contemporary magazines, scissors, glue, colored markers and a piece of posterboard for each group. See Activity 3 (p. 35).

UNIT OVERVIEW

PURPOSE

Many Americans believe that thinner is better. People with eating disorders believe it so deeply that weight and dieting success become the measure of their self-esteem. These people become trapped in a cycle of repeated, ritualistic and rigid behavior focused on food and eating. The activities in this unit provide students with the opportunities to understand and analyze the characteristics of eating disorders and how those behaviors are related to body image and self-esteem.

MAIN POINTS

✳ Adolescent preoccupation with physical and biological body changes is normal.

✳ Some dieting behaviors among adolescents may be considered normal, but obsession with thinness, body weight or food may indicate a severe psychological problem that requires professional help.

✳ Overemphasis on thinness during adolescence may contribute to the increasing incidence of anorexia nervosa and bulimia in the United States.

✳ Eating disorders occur in epidemic proportions among females.

✳ These eating disorders affect males to a smaller degree.

✳ Individuals with eating disorders tend to believe that their self-worth is tied to body weight and dieting success.

REVIEW

To increase your understanding of eating disorders, review **Adolescents and Eating Disorders** *Instant Expert* (p. 38) and **Check Your Knowledge Key** (p. 45).

VOCABULARY

amenorrhea—The absence or cessation of menstruation.

anorexia nervosa—Eating disorder characterized by self-imposed starvation and refusal to maintain a minimally normal weight.

binge—Eating an extraordinarily large amount of food at one time.

bulimia—Eating disorder characterized by repeated episodes of binge eating followed by purging behaviors such as self-induced vomiting, misuse of laxatives or diuretics, fasting and excessive exercise.

cathartic—Stronger, faster-acting laxative.

diuretic—A drug that helps relieve the body of excess water.

dysmorphophobia—An obsession with a particular body flaw.

eating disorder—A health-threatening upset in patterns of food consumption.

fast—To go without food.

laxative—A substance that loosens the bowels and relieves constipation.

purgative—Stronger, faster-acting laxative.

purging—Attempts to rid the body of food, including self-induced vomiting and laxative or diuretic abuse.

starvation—Dying from lack of food.

trigger—An event that sets off a certain behavior cycle.

1. WHAT DO YOU KNOW?

5 minutes

MATERIALS
◆ Check Your Knowledge (3.1)

MEETING STUDENT NEEDS

Students should be assured from the beginning that they have the right to pass during any discussion or activity that involves personal opinions, feelings or experiences. Be sensitive to student feelings and provide privacy for personal assessments. Be prepared to refer students to professional help or counseling for problem eating behaviors or excessive concerns about body image.

A SELF-ASSESSMENT ACTIVITY

Students take pretest

Distribute the **Check Your Knowledge** activity sheet and have students complete it. This activity sheet measures how much students know about eating disorders. Explain that at the end of the unit they will take the survey again to see how much they've learned.

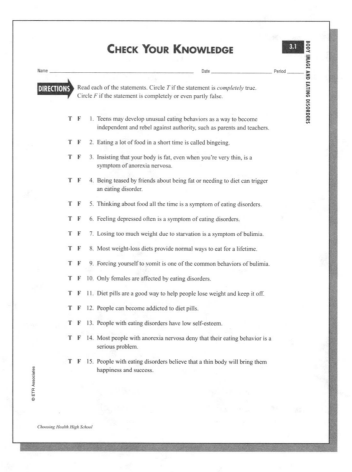

CHECK YOUR KNOWLEDGE   3.1

Name _____ Date _____ Period _____

DIRECTIONS Read each of the statements. Circle *T* if the statement is *completely* true. Circle *F* if the statement is completely or even partly false.

T F   1. Teens may develop unusual eating behaviors as a way to become independent and rebel against authority, such as parents and teachers.

T F   2. Eating a lot of food in a short time is called bingeing.

T F   3. Insisting that your body is fat, even when you're very thin, is a symptom of anorexia nervosa.

T F   4. Being teased by friends about being fat or needing to diet can trigger an eating disorder.

T F   5. Thinking about food all the time is a symptom of eating disorders.

T F   6. Feeling depressed often is a symptom of eating disorders.

T F   7. Losing too much weight due to starvation is a symptom of bulimia.

T F   8. Most weight-loss diets provide normal ways to eat for a lifetime.

T F   9. Forcing yourself to vomit is one of the common behaviors of bulimia.

T F 10. Only females are affected by eating disorders.

T F 11. Diet pills are a good way to help people lose weight and keep it off.

T F 12. People can become addicted to diet pills.

T F 13. People with eating disorders have low self-esteem.

T F 14. Most people with anorexia nervosa deny that their eating behavior is a serious problem.

T F 15. People with eating disorders believe that a thin body will bring them happiness and success.

© ETR Associates

Choosing Health High School

BODY IMAGE AND EATING DISORDERS

2. LEARNING ABOUT EATING DISORDERS

⟨ A SMALL GROUP ACTIVITY ⟩

Groups study eating disorders

Divide the class into 4 groups and distribute a different student reading page to each group—*What Causes Eating Disorders?, What Is Anorexia Nervosa?, What Is Bulimia?, Drugs and Eating Disorders.* Explain the group assignment:

- Read and discuss the information.
- Prepare a class presentation on the topic.

Provide blank transparencies or butcher paper and encourage students to make lists of symptoms and other important points to use during the group presentations.

(continued…)

45 minutes

MATERIALS

- What Causes Eating Disorders? (3.2)
- What Is Anorexia Nervosa? (3.3)
- What Is Bulimia? (3.4)
- Drugs and Eating Disorders (3.5)
- butcher paper or blank transparencies

WHAT CAUSES EATING DISORDERS? `3.2`

STUDENT READING

Many teenagers believe that dieting [is a] normal way to eat. Magazines, billbo[ards,] television shows and commercials all [give] the message that being thin leads to h[appiness,] success, self-confidence and respect.

People with eating disorders belie[ve these] messages. They spend a lot of their tim[e] thinking about what they eat and how [they look.] They focus so much on their appearan[ce they] don't develop confidence and abilities [in other areas.]

PSYCHOLOGICAL FACTORS

People who have eating disorders a[lways have a] negative body image. They tend to ha[ve low self-] esteem and feel inadequate. They ofte[n try] to prove they are good enough, becau[se] they're afraid they aren't. They tend t[o be] competitive and ambitious. They wan[t to be perfect.] They think that if they are thin, they w[ill be] popular, successful and confident.

FAMILY PROBLEMS

Some teens use eating disorders a[s a way to] remain dependent on their parents. Th[ey are] afraid to grow up and leave the safety [of] their families. Others use their unusua[l] behaviors as a way to assert their inde[pendence or] rebel against family standards.

An eating disorder can be a way t[o rebel] against strict parents. In some familie[s, a teen] feels he or she has to take care of the [family and] does not want this unfair responsibili[ty.]

LIFESTYLE FACTORS

People with eating disorders tend [to be] very assertive. They usually don't han[dle stress] well. They often don't have goals (oth[er than] weight loss) that can help them feel i[mportant] and self-confident.

They may have friends who are al[so] concerned about physical appearance. Many dancers, actresses, models, gym [attendants, sorority members and jock[eys have] eating disorders.

Choosing Health High School

WHAT IS ANOREXIA NERVOSA? `3.3`

STUDENT READING

Anorexia nervosa is a serious eatin[g disorder.] People with this disorder say they feel [that] parts of their body are fat, even if they [weigh] less than is normal or healthy.

Some people are just naturally ver[y thin. That] doesn't mean they are anorexic. What [sets people] with anorexia nervosa apart are their a[ttitudes about] food and their desire to be even thinn[er. People] with anorexia nervosa are very concer[ned about] their body size and are usually unhapp[y with some] feature of their physical appearance. T[hey spend a] lot of time thinking about eating, food [and] body image.

They may count calories, weigh th[emselves] many times a day and go on strict diet[s, even if they] are very thin. They may feel uncomfo[rtable] eating a normal or even a very small [meal. They] may think of foods as good or bad. Th[ey may] judge how well they control their eati[ng and] measure their success in terms of how [much] they can lose.

People with anorexia nervosa usu[ally control their] weight by fasting and/or reducing the [amount of] food they eat and exercising a lot. Som[e...]

Choosing Health High School

WHAT IS BULIMIA? `3.4`

STUDENT READING

Bulimia is an eating disorder that [involves] bingeing and purging. Bingeing (bing[ing) means] eating a large amount of food in a sho[rt period of] time. Purging refers to trying to get ri[d of food] that's been eaten by vomiting or using [laxatives or] diuretics.

People with bulimia often feel the[y have no] control during binges. They find it har[d to resist the] urge to binge or to stop once they've s[tarted. They] also may try other ways to prevent we[ight gain,] including strict diets, diet aids, fasts o[r excessive] exercise.

Some people with bulimia may pl[an their] binges. They buy sweet, high-calorie [food to eat] during the binge. This food may also [be eaten] quickly, without a lot of chewing, suc[h as ice] cream. The binge is usually kept hidde[n from] others. Once the binge has begun, the [person may] look for more food to eat when the foo[d for] the binge is gone.

A binge usually ends when the bin[ger's stomach] starts to hurt or if someone interrupts. [After] bingeing, many bulimics make themse[lves vomit to] purge the food. Vomiting usually redu[ces...]

Choosing Health High School

DRUGS AND EATING DISORDERS `3.5`

STUDENT READING

People with eating disorders may abuse several types of drugs.

LAXATIVES

Laxatives seem to move food through the body more rapidly. They may relieve stomach bloating and pain after a binge. But they don't prevent the calories in food from being absorbed. Any weight loss is due mostly to loss of water and minerals and is only temporary.

Misuse of laxatives is harmful:

- They upset the body's mineral balance.
- They lead to dehydration (not enough water in the cells of the body).
- They damage the lining of the digestive tract.
- They let the digestive tract get lazy. Someone who uses laxatives regularly may become constipated without them.

DIURETICS

Diuretics, or water pills, help the body get rid of excess water by increasing the amount of urine. They can cause sudden weight loss. But they also cause dehydration. Diuretics are dangerous. They increase the loss of important minerals—calcium, potassium, magnesium and zinc—from the body. In a rebound effect, they can also cause the body to retain salt and water, and make it more sensitive to diet changes.

IPECAC SYRUP

Ipecac syrup is taken to cause vomiting. It has been linked to the deaths of several people with eating disorders. The active ingredient (emetine) can build up in body tissues and cause muscle or heart weakness. Ipecac is toxic (poisonous), whether taken in a large amount or small amounts that build up over time.

DIET PILLS

Pills are often taken to help with weight loss. The best known pills are Dexedrine and Benzedrine. These require a prescription from a doctor. But the FDA prohibits doctors from prescribing these drugs for weight loss.

Some over-the-counter drugs, available without a prescription, can also be used to temporarily reduce appetite. But usually the appetite returns to normal after a week or so, and the lost weight is gained back. Then the user has the problem of trying to get off the drug without gaining more weight.

Drugs do not really help people lose weight and keep it off. They can be addictive, and lead to dangerous physical problems if misused.

Choosing Health High School

2. LEARNING ABOUT EATING DISORDERS

CONTINUED

COMMUNITY LINK

Assign students to research the services available in your community to help young people with eating disorders. Ask students to make a poster with phone numbers as a resource to post in the classroom.

Groups present

Have groups make their presentations. Discuss eating disorders, using **Adolescents and Eating Disorders** *Instant Expert* as a guide. Cover any points groups may have overlooked in their presentations.

Ongoing Assessment Look for students to demonstrate general understanding that eating disorders:

- are serious and complex and can result in death
- are influenced by feelings of low self-esteem or other mental health issues
- need treatment

3. INFLUENCES ON EATING DISORDERS

Groups create collages

Put students in groups of 4 or 5. Distribute a piece of posterboard to each group, and make scissors, glue, tape, colored markers and magazines available. Explain the group assignment:

- Use pictures from magazines or your own drawings to develop a collage that represents factors that influence body image and eating disorders.
- Label each factor that relates to the characteristics associated with the eating disorders discussed in class.
- Prepare to present your collage to the class, explaining the images you used.

Groups present

Have groups present and explain their collages. Post the collages in the classroom.

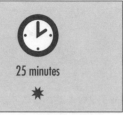

25 minutes

MATERIALS

- posterboard
- magazines
- scissors, glue and tape
- colored markers

EXTEND THE LEARNING

Students can read stories and books about people with eating disorders and their experiences. Possible subjects include Princess Diana, Karen Carpenter, Cherry Boone, Jane Fonda and Cathy Rigby-McCoy.

EVALUATION

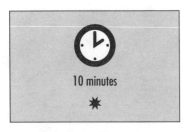

10 minutes

REVIEW

◆ Check Your Knowledge *Key*
    (p. 45)

MATERIALS

◆ Check Your Knowledge (3.1)

OBJECTIVE 1

Students will be able to:

> **Identify the characteristics of eating disorders.**

Distribute a second copy of the **Check Your Knowledge** activity sheet and have students complete it.

CRITERIA

Review the correct answers on the activity sheet with the class, using the **Check Your Knowledge** *Key* as a guide. Have students write a paragraph comparing their scores on the pretest and posttest.

(continued...)

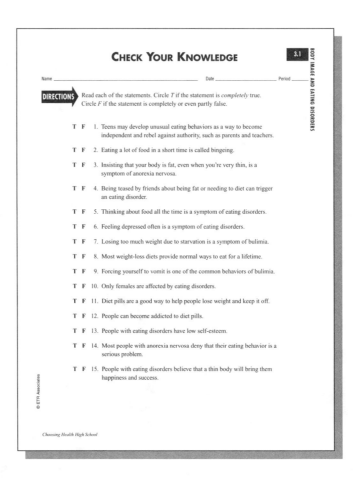

EVALUATION

OBJECTIVE 2

Students will be able to:

> **Explain the relationship between eating disorders and body image.**

Have students write a paragraph that answers the question: How are eating disorders related to body image?

CRITERIA

Assess students' ability to describe the relationship between eating disorders and body image. Look for students to describe characteristics of eating disorders that relate to distorted body image. See the **Adolescents and Eating Disorders** *Instant Expert* for evaluation criteria.

20 minutes

REVIEW

♦ Adolescents and Eating Disorders *Instant Expert* (p. 38)

ADOLESCENTS AND EATING DISORDERS

In the United States, magazines, billboards, movies, television shows and commercials all seem to send a message that being thin leads to happiness and success. People with eating disorders believe these messages and spend much of their time and energy thinking about what they eat and how they look. Eating disorders are serious illnesses. They may have severe and even life-threatening health consequences.

Eating disorders are more prevalent in industrialized societies in which there is an abundance of food, and in which, especially for females, there is cultural pressure to be thin. There are at least 8 million victims of eating disorders in the United States. As many as 6% of the serious cases die. Eating disorders affect 10–15% of adolescent girls. Although 90% of the victims are women, male cases are being reported with increasing frequency.

TEENS AND WEIGHT LOSS

Many teenagers believe that dieting is the normal way to eat. In 1966, as many as 70% of high school girls were reported to be unhappy with their bodies and wanted to lose weight. Twenty years later, 63% of high school girls indicated that they were dieting on the day of the survey. According to the Centers for Disease Control and Prevention (1995), 40% of students in grades 9–12 were attempting weight loss. In the same study, one third of all students thought they were overweight.

Females were more likely than males to identify themselves as being overweight. Methods of weight loss used by adolescent girls include diet pills, fasting and crash diets. Their sources of information about weight control and dieting tend to be the mass media, family members and athletic coaches. Teachers and the school nurse are rarely consulted.

Teenagers are particularly vulnerable to eating disorders. Problems around food and eating usually begin in the early to late teens. Anorexia nervosa and bulimia are the most serious eating disorders afflicting today's teenagers.

SYMPTOMS OF ANOREXIA NERVOSA

Individuals who suffer from anorexia nervosa are underweight—less than 85% of the weight considered normal for their age and height. Individuals with this disorder have an intense fear of gaining weight or becoming fat. This fear is not alleviated by weight loss, and often increases even as body weight continues to decrease.

Anorexics' perception of their body weight and shape are distorted. Some feel globally overweight; others realize they are thin but are concerned that certain parts of their bodies, particularly the abdomen, buttocks or thighs, are "too fat."

(continued...)

ADOLESCENTS AND EATING DISORDERS

They may count calories, weigh themselves many times a day and go on strict diets or fast, even if they are already thin. They may think of foods as good or bad. They may also judge how well they control their eating habits. Weight loss is viewed as an impressive achievement and a sign of self-discipline; weight gain is viewed as failure.

Anorexics usually lose weight by reducing the amount of food they eat and exercising excessively. They may feel uncomfortable after eating a normal-sized or even a very small meal. At least 40% of people with anorexia nervosa also suffer from bulimia.

Peculiar behaviors around food are common in people with anorexia nervosa. They often fix very special meals for others, but limit themselves to a few low-calorie foods. They may have special rituals around food, hide it or throw it away. Some may feel compelled to wash their hands frequently. Most people with anorexia nervosa deny that they have a problem with food.

Amenorrhea, the stopping of the regular menstrual cycle, is a possible consequence of the extreme weight loss. If anorexia nervosa begins before puberty, menarche may be delayed by the illness.

The average age of onset for anorexia nervosa is 14 years, but tends to peak at 17 and 18 years of age. Onset is often associated with a stressful life event, such as leaving home for college. Anorexia nervosa is more common among people who have sisters and mothers who have the disorder.

Many people have only one episode of anorexia nervosa and then return to normal eating patterns and weight. But in some cases, weight loss is so severe that the person has to be hospitalized to prevent death by starvation. Studies indicate that 5–18% of people with this eating disorder die.

SYMPTOMS OF BULIMIA

People with bulimia are typically within the normal weight range for their age and height, although some may be slightly underweight or overweight. Whatever they weigh, they are very concerned about their weight and body shape.

(continued...)

ADOLESCENTS AND EATING DISORDERS

Bulimia is characterized by bingeing and purging. Bingeing (binge eating) is eating a large amount (more than most people would eat in a similar circumstance) of food in a short period of time (less than 2 hours). Purging refers to trying to get rid of the food that's been eaten by vomiting or using laxatives, enemas or diuretics. To be diagnosed with bulimia, the binge eating and purging must occur on average at least twice a week for 3 months.

People with bulimia often feel they are out of control during binges. They may have difficulty resisting the urge to binge or difficulty stopping once a binge has begun. They also may try other ways to prevent weight gain, including diet aids, strict diets, fasts or lots of exercise.

Some people with bulimia plan their eating binges. Often the food they buy to eat during a binge is sweet and high in calories with little nutrient density. It may also be easy to eat quickly, without a lot of chewing, such as ice cream. The binge is usually kept hidden from others. Once the binge has begun, the person may look for more food to eat when the food that started the binge is gone.

A binge usually ends when the person's stomach starts to hurt or if someone interrupts. About 80–90% of individuals with bulimia induce vomiting after binge eating. Vomiting usually reduces the stomach pain. Then the person either starts eating again or ends the binge. Sometimes a binge ends with the person going to sleep.

Some people with bulimia may have the urge to vomit. They will binge in order to vomit or will vomit after eating a small amount of food. Although a binge may seem enjoyable at the time, the person often feels depressed afterwards. Some people with bulimia may fast for a day or more or exercise excessively in an attempt to compensate for the binge.

Binges usually alternate with periods of normal eating or with periods of normal eating and fasting. When the problem gets worse, the victim may either binge or fast with no periods of normal eating. Weight may change often due to the alternating binges and fasts.

The problem usually begins in adolescence or early adulthood. Approximately 1–3% of adolescent and young adult females have this eating disorder. The rate among males is about one-tenth of that in females.

(continued...)

ADOLESCENTS AND EATING DISORDERS

Bulimia can lead to numerous physical problems and complications. Repeated vomiting commonly causes gastritis, an inflammation of the stomach lining, and can injure the esophagus. Acid from the stomach irritates and inflames the membrane that lines the esophagus, sometimes causing scarring and narrowing. The physical stress of vomiting can cause tears in the lining of the esophagus, leading to massive bleeding or even rupture. These problems can be life-threatening.

Chronic vomiting increases the acidity of the mouth and results in erosion of the tooth enamel and dentin. Lung complications can also occur when self-induced vomiting leads to aspiration of food particles, gastric acid and bacteria.

Laxative abuse commonly results in injury to the intestines, particularly the colon. Damage to the intestinal lining may lead to ulcers and produce bloody stools. Phenolphthalein, an ingredient found in most over-the-counter laxatives, may cause sores in the skin and hyperpigmentation (brown or gray spots).

Fasting, vomiting and other forms of purging result in loss of fluids and crucial minerals from the body. Chronic dehydration and low potassium levels can lead to kidney stones and even kidney failure.

Loss of body acids as a result of frequent vomiting leads to high alkali levels in the blood and body tissues. This may cause weakness, constipation and tiredness. Severe alkalosis and potassium deficiency can lead to an uneven heart rate or sudden death.

INFLUENCES ON EATING DISORDERS

A variety of factors influence the development of eating disorders, including:
- psychological factors
- family problems
- lifestyle factors
- biological factors
- nutrition

Psychological factors: People with eating disorders are unable to realistically assess their own weight. They tend to have lower self-esteem, a more negative body image, and more feelings of inadequacy, self-doubt, anxiety and depression. They may be particularly sensitive to external pressures to be a certain way or to do certain things and tend to look for approval from others.

(continued...)

Adolescents and Eating Disorders

People who have eating disorders are often competitive, ambitious and perfectionistic. Yet they also suffer from fears of failing or proving inadequate. They equate being thin with being happy, popular, successful and self-confident.

Family problems: Some teens use eating disorders as an excuse to remain dependent on their parents; they may be afraid to grow up and leave the safety of school and their families. Others, especially those with overly protective parents, may use their unusual food behaviors as a way to assert their independence and rebel against family standards.

An eating disorder can be a symbolic protest against parents the teen thinks are too strict. In other families, the teen feels he or she has to take care of the parents and does not want this unfair responsibility.

Lifestyle factors: People with eating disorders tend to not be very assertive. They usually don't handle stress well. They often don't have important goals (other than weight loss) that can help them feel independent and self-confident.

They may have friends who are also very concerned about physical appearance and thinness. Many dancers, actresses, models, gymnasts, flight attendants, sorority members and jockeys have eating disorders.

Biological factors: Some people may be more likely than others to develop an eating disorder. Biological factors may be related to alcoholism or depression or both. People with certain types of eating disorders may abuse alcohol and other drugs.

There is an increased risk of anorexia nervosa and bulimia for first-degree biological relatives of individuals with the disorder. A familial tendency toward obesity may exist for individuals with bulimia.

Nutrition: Dieting or limiting eating over a long period of time can cause body processes to be out of balance. These changes in the body can lead to eating disorders. However, most physical problems are results, not causes, of eating disorders.

Poor nutrition causes changes in the way the body uses calories from food. These changes make it harder to lose weight and easier to gain it. The frustration this causes can lead people to overeat (binge), then try to get rid of the food by purging. Purging, especially vomiting, decreases the basal metabolic rate (the body's use of calories to maintain body functions) and decreases the number of calories the body needs. These results can make the problem even worse.

(continued...)

ADOLESCENTS AND EATING DISORDERS

TRIGGERS FOR EATING DISORDERS

Many of the factors that contribute to eating disorders can exist for years before anything happens. Then something may set off a cycle of strict dieting or bingeing and purging. The event that sets off this cycle is called a *trigger*.

Trigger incidents are usually problems the person is not prepared to handle. Triggers can include losses, such as death, divorce or leaving home; school pressures; a long-distance move; or the break-up of an important relationship. Many teens with eating disorders report that teasing from their peers or other comments about their bodies made them decide they were fat and needed to diet.

Many people with eating disorders are also victims of rape, incest, molestation, verbal abuse and neglect. Because they don't know how to express their fear, rage, confusion and need for help, they turn to or away from food. They may use food for comfort, or they may go on strict diets to help them feel in control of something in their lives.

DRUGS AND EATING DISORDERS

A variety of drugs can be misused by people with eating disorders. These drugs don't really help people lose weight and keep it off, and they can be dangerously addictive. Drugs most commonly used in this manner include:

- laxatives
- diuretics
- ipecac syrup
- diet pills

Laxatives: Laxatives seem to move food through the body more rapidly. They may relieve stomach bloating and pain after a binge. However, they don't prevent the calories in food from being absorbed. Any weight loss is due mostly to loss of water and minerals in the bowel movement and is temporary.

Misuse of laxatives has harmful effects, including:

- upset of the body's mineral balance
- dehydration
- damage to the lining of the digestive tract
- digestive tract may become dependent on laxatives to avoid constipation

(continued...)

ADOLESCENTS AND EATING DISORDERS

Diuretics: Diuretics, or water pills, increase the amount of urine excreted from the body. They can cause sudden weight loss and dehydration. Diuretics are dangerous because they can increase the loss of important minerals—calcium, potassium, magnesium and zinc—from the body. In a rebound effect, they can also cause the body to retain salt and water, making it more sensitive to diet changes.

Ipecac syrup: A few individuals consume ipecac syrup to induce vomiting. It has been linked to the deaths of several people with eating disorders. The active ingredient (emetine) can build up in body tissues and cause muscle or heart weakness. Ipecac is toxic, whether taken in a large amount or small amounts that build up over time.

Diet pills: Diet pills, such as Fastin, increase metabolism and reduce appetite. Dexedrine and Benzedrine are also taken to help with weight loss. Dexedrine and Benzedrine require a prescription from a doctor; however, the FDA prohibits doctors from prescribing these drugs for weight loss. They are stimulant drugs used to treat depression, narcolepsy, central nervous system disorders and Attention Deficit Hyperactivity Disorder.

Some over-the-counter drugs, available without a prescription, can also be used to reduce the appetite. The reduction of appetite is only temporary, however. Usually appetite returns to normal after a week or so, and the lost weight is regained. Then the user has the problem of trying to get off the drug without gaining more weight.

CHECK YOUR KNOWLEDGE

KEY

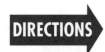 **DIRECTIONS** Read each of the statements. Circle *T* if the statement is *completely* true. Circle *F* if the statement is completely or even partly false.

(T) F 1. Teens may develop unusual eating behaviors as a way to become independent and rebel against authority, such as parents and teachers.

(T) F 2. Eating a lot of food in a short time is called bingeing.

(T) F 3. Insisting that your body is fat, even when you're very thin, is a symptom of anorexia nervosa.

(T) F 4. Being teased by friends about being fat or needing to diet can trigger an eating disorder.

(T) F 5. Thinking about food all the time is a symptom of eating disorders.

(T) F 6. Feeling depressed often is a symptom of eating disorders.

T (F) 7. Losing too much weight due to starvation is a symptom of bulimia.

T (F) 8. Most weight-loss diets provide normal ways to eat for a lifetime.

(T) F 9. Forcing yourself to vomit is one of the common behaviors of bulimia.

T (F) 10. Only females are affected by eating disorders.

T (F) 11. Diet pills are a good way to help people lose weight and keep it off.

(T) F 12. People can become addicted to diet pills.

(T) F 13. People with eating disorders have low self-esteem.

(T) F 14. Most people with anorexia nervosa deny that their eating behavior is a serious problem.

T F 15. People with eating disorders believe that a thin body will bring them happiness and success.

© ETR Associates

HELP FOR EATING DISORDERS

TIME

2–3 periods

ACTIVITIES

1. Circles of Sharing

2. What's Normal?

3. Help for Eating Disorders

4. What's Eating You?

HELP FOR EATING DISORDERS

OBJECTIVES

Students will be able to:

> 1. Illustrate prevention behaviors for eating disorders.

> 2. Differentiate between normal teenage eating behaviors and eating disorder behaviors.

GETTING STARTED

Have:

- butcher paper or posterboard
- markers
- art supplies

Copy for each student:

- Privacy Circles (4.1)
- Problems Eating You? (4.4)

Make transparency of:

- Privacy Circles (4.1)
- Prevention Pointers (4.2)
- Help for Eating Disorders (4.3)

UNIT OVERVIEW

PURPOSE

The best treatment for eating disorders is prevention. Early detection of a possible problem and prompt, competent treatment is important. Activities in this unit help students recognize if they, or someone they know, might have an eating disorder and analyze whom they can talk to about possible problems.

MAIN POINTS

* Individuals with eating disorders must face the problem before they can get help.
* The most difficult factor in the treatment of eating disorders is overcoming body-image distortions and the fear of becoming fat.
* Treatment needs to focus more on *attitudes* about eating, weight and body shape than on eating habits.

REVIEW

To increase your understanding of treatments for eating disorders, review Overcoming Eating Disorders *Instant Expert* (p. 57).

VOCABULARY

confide—To share sensitive or personal information with another person.

normal—Conforming with an accepted standard; natural.

prevention—Hindering or stopping something from happening or existing.

privacy—One's private life; those things kept secret or closely guarded.

stress—The feeling of being under pressure.

stressor—Anything that triggers a stress response.

therapy—The treatment of a physical or mental disorder by medical or psychological means.

treatment—A course of action to stop a disease.

1. CIRCLES OF SHARING

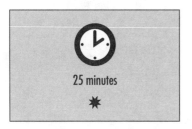

25 minutes

MATERIALS

◆ Privacy Circles (4.1)
◆ transparency of Privacy Circles (4.1)

Students identify confidants

Distribute the **Privacy Circles** activity sheet. Ask students to identify in the center circle the person in whom they feel most comfortable confiding, the person in their life whom they feel they can tell anything. Students can use initials or a secret code to indicate this person.

Have students identify the second most likely person to whom they would confide in the second circle from the center. Have them continue filling in the circles. As they move outward from the center, each of the circles represents someone in whom they would be less likely to confide.

Display the transparency of the **Privacy Circles** activity sheet and demonstrate the process of putting initials in each of the circles.

(continued...)

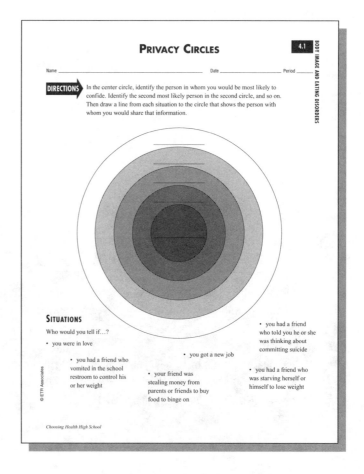

1. CIRCLES OF SHARING

(CONTINUED)

Students examine situations

Ask students to look at each of the situations listed on the activity sheet. Have them draw a line from each situation to the circle that indicates the person with whom they would share that information or problem. Demonstrate on the **Privacy Circles** transparency.

Discuss students' work

Ask students:

- Were there any situations you felt you could share (would not mind telling) with anyone in any of your circles or people outside (not listed in) the circles?
- Were there situations you would not share with anyone, even the person in the innermost privacy circle?
- Which situations were more private to you?
- Why are some situations more private to some people than to others?

Review each of the situations. Ask students where they could find help if they needed it for themselves, friends or family members.

Ongoing Assessment) Look for students to draw conclusions about the difficulty of sharing information about an eating disorder.

MEETING STUDENT NEEDS

Remind students that they should not be disclosing personal information. This activity is for their own self-awareness. Specific personal information should not be discussed with the class.

---

2. WHAT'S NORMAL?

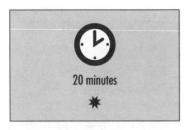

20 minutes

MATERIALS
- butcher paper
- markers

Groups analyze eating behaviors

Divide the class into groups of 4 or 5. Give each group a piece of butcher paper and a marking pen. Explain the group assignment:

- Divide the butcher paper into 2 columns.
- Label the first column "Normal Eating Behavior" and the other "Eating Disorders."
- In the Normal Eating column, list behaviors that are normal eating behaviors.
- In the Eating Disorders column, list behaviors that indicate an eating disorder.

Groups report

Label another piece of butcher paper with the column headings "Normal Eating Behavior" and "Eating Disorders" or write the headings on the board. Have groups share their lists with the class. As groups report, compile their lists.

Discuss normal teenage dieting and weight control behaviors versus eating disorders, using the Normal or Not? section of the **Overcoming Eating Disorders** *Instant Expert* as a guide. Add to the lists any other eating behaviors that come up in discussion.

Ongoing Assessment Look for students' understanding that being obsessed with food; eating very small amounts (little or nothing); and bingeing on large amounts of food, especially within a *planned* period of time, followed by purging are *not* normal eating behaviors.

3. HELP FOR EATING DISORDERS

Discuss prevention pointers

Display the Prevention Pointers transparency and discuss each step. Stress that, because eating disorders can be very difficult to treat, prevention is very important.

Identify resources

Display the Help for Eating Disorders transparency. Explain that these organizations offer help to people with eating disorders. Answer any questions students may have about treatment of eating disorders, using the Overcoming Eating Disorders *Instant Expert* as a guide.

15 minutes

MATERIALS

- transparency of Prevention Pointers (4.2)
- transparency of Help for Eating Disorders (4.3)

COMMUNITY LINK

Students can prepare oral reports on a referral or treatment resource for eating disorders in your community.

Have students write to the organizations on the **Help for Eating Disorders** list and report on their findings. Information to obtain might include the name and address of resource, type of treatment used, whether treatment is inpatient or outpatient, and cost of treatment.

PREVENTION POINTERS
4.2 | BODY IMAGE AND EATING DISORDERS

- **Learn to like yourself, just as you are.**

- **Set realistic goals for yourself.**

- **Ask for support ment from frien when life is stres**

- **Learn the basics and exercise.**

- **If you want to lo to a doctor or a registered dietit in weight contro**

- **Seek adult help or a friend has a problem.**

© ETR Associates

Choosing Health High School

HELP FOR EATING DISORDERS
4.3 | BODY IMAGE AND EATING DISORDERS

NATIONAL NONPROFIT EATING DISORDERS ORGANIZATIONS

AABA
American Anorexia/Bulimia Association
418 E. 76th Street
New York, NY 10021
(212) 734-1114

ABC
Anorexia Bulimia Care, Inc.
545 Concord Avenue
Cambridge, MA 02138-1122
(617) 492-7670

ANAD
National Association of Anorexia
Nervosa and Associated Disorders
P.O. Box 7
Highland Park, IL 60035
(847) 831-3438

ANRED
Anorexia Nervosa and Related Eating
Disorders
P.O. Box 5102
Eugene, OR 97405
(503) 344-1144

EDAP
Eating Disorders Awareness
and Prevention
255 Alhambra Circle, #321
Coral Gables, FL 33134
(305) 444-3731

F.E.E.D.
Foundation for Education about Eating
Disorders
5238 Duvall Drive
Bethesda, MD 20816

IAEDP
International Association of Eating
Disorders Professionals
123 NW 13th Street, #206
Boca Raton, FL 33432-1618
(800) 800-8126

NAAS
National Anorexic Aid Society
1925 E. Dublin-Granville Road
Columbus, OH 43229
(614) 436-1112

OA
Overeaters Anonymous Headquarters
World Services Office
P.O. Box 92870
Los Angeles, CA 90009
(310) 618-8835

© ETR Associates

Choosing Health High School

---

4. WHAT'S EATING YOU?

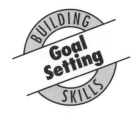

20 minutes

✳

MATERIALS

♦ Problems Eating You? (4.4)

✳

MEETING STUDENT NEEDS

The questions on the **Problems Eating You?** activity sheet may alert a student to a possible eating disorder problem or poor self-image. Explain that a yes answer to 1 or more of the questions indicates a need to talk to a trusted adult about eating disorders. Offer to speak to students with concerns or refer them to the school counselor or nurse.

✳

Students assess possible eating disorders

Distribute the **Problems Eating You?** activity sheet. Ask students to think about a friend or family member they might be concerned about and complete the questionnaire for this person. They should not use the person's name. Students can also complete this assignment using a fictional person.

Students write letters

Have students write a letter to a friend (real or fictional) who is showing signs of an eating disorder. Tell them to be sure to include the following points:

- Identify the observed behaviors.
- Identify where the friend can get help.
- Show genuine concern and caring for the friend.

Ongoing Assessment Look for student letters to identify specific behaviors that may indicate a problem. Letters should also include a way to get help and express concern for the person.

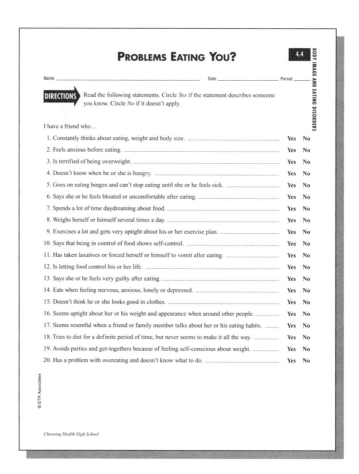

PROBLEMS EATING YOU? **4.4**

BODY IMAGE AND EATING DISORDERS

Name _____ Date _____ Period ____

DIRECTIONS Read the following statements. Circle *Yes* if the statement describes someone you know. Circle *No* if it doesn't apply.

I have a friend who…

1. Constantly thinks about eating, weight and body size. .... Yes No
2. Feels anxious before eating. .... Yes No
3. Is terrified of being overweight. .... Yes No
4. Doesn't know when he or she is hungry. .... Yes No
5. Goes on eating binges and can't stop eating until she or he feels sick. ...... Yes No
6. Says she or he feels bloated or uncomfortable after eating. .... Yes No
7. Spends a lot of time daydreaming about food. .... Yes No
8. Weighs herself or himself several times a day. .... Yes No
9. Exercises a lot and gets very uptight about his or her exercise plan. .... Yes No
10. Says that being in control of food shows self-control. .... Yes No
11. Has taken laxatives or forced herself or himself to vomit after eating. ...... Yes No
12. Is letting food control his or her life. .... Yes No
13. Says she or he feels very guilty after eating. .... Yes No
14. Eats when feeling nervous, anxious, lonely or depressed. .... Yes No
15. Doesn't think he or she looks good in clothes. .... Yes No
16. Seems uptight about her or his weight and appearance when around other people. ...... Yes No
17. Seems resentful when a friend or family member talks about her or his eating habits. ...... Yes No
18. Tries to diet for a definite period of time, but never seems to make it all the way. ...... Yes No
19. Avoids parties and get-togethers because of feeling self-conscious about weight. ...... Yes No
20. Has a problem with overeating and doesn't know what to do. .... Yes No

© ETR Associates

Choosing Health High School

EVALUATION

OBJECTIVE 1

Students will be able to:

> **Illustrate prevention behaviors for eating disorders.**

Make art supplies and posterboard available. Have students design a poster that illustrates at least 1 of the prevention behaviors for eating disorders. Encourage students to be creative and to emphasize the positive.

CRITERIA

Assess students' ability to present at least 1 of the following key prevention points:

- Learn to like yourself, just as you are.
- Set realistic goals for yourself.
- Ask for support and encouragement from friends and family when life is stressful.
- Learn the basics of good nutrition and exercise.
- If you want to lose weight, talk to a doctor or a professional, registered dietitian who specializes in weight control.
- Seek adult help if you suspect you or a friend has an eating disorder.

(continued...)

20 minutes

MATERIALS

- ◆ art supplies
- ◆ posterboard or butcher paper

EVALUATION

25 minutes

※

OBJECTIVE 2

Students will be able to:

> **Differentiate between normal teenage eating behaviors and eating disorder behaviors.**

Have students write fictional case studies about 2 teenagers. One of the case studies should describe a teen who potentially has an eating disorder and the other should describe normal teenage eating behaviors.

CRITERIA

Assess students' ability to differentiate between normal teenage eating behaviors and behaviors that indicate a possible eating disorder.

Normal eating behaviors include:

- Eats reasonable portions of foods.
- Usually eats balanced meals with a variety of foods.
- Eats the same types and amounts of food whether eating with others or alone.
- Eats enough to maintain a reasonable body weight.
- Exercises regularly for fitness.
- Sometimes eats as a response to stress.
- Sometimes diets in response to body image concerns.

Behaviors that indicate a possible eating disorder include:

- When eating with others, eats nothing or plays with food.
- Uses purging or vomiting to get rid of food.
- Binges—eats large amounts of food within a short time.
- Plans eating binges.
- Exercises to be slim and to use calories; may exercise too much.
- Prefers to eat alone.
- Appears to be obsessed with thoughts of food.

OVERCOMING EATING DISORDERS

The first step in overcoming an eating disorder is recognizing the problem—perhaps the most difficult aspect of these secretive disorders. Individuals with eating disorders cannot get help unless they realize they have a problem.

Recognizing and sharing with another that you suspect a problem can be difficult. But it is essential before an individual can obtain help for the eating disorder.

THE STRESS CONNECTION

The use and abuse of food as a response to stress is common among high school and college students. Because the adolescent years can be critical in forming lifetime habits, this is the ideal time for teachers, counselors and parents to help young people learn healthy ways to cope with feelings of stress and/or failure. This is also a critical time to address feelings of guilt concerning food abuse and the desire to be thin.

Research done by Dona M. Kagan in 1987 indicated that compulsive eating among young women appeared to be a response to environmental stress. Among young men it was more likely to indicate deficiencies in the family system. Among more than 2,000 high school and college-age women studied, disordered eating habits were consistently associated with feelings of stress, failure and low self-esteem. Males who tended to eat compulsively saw their families as relatively uncohesive and rigid. They were dissatisfied with their family life and reported cold relationships with their parents.

Adolescents need to identify other means of releasing stress besides overeating. They also need to understand that thinness and weight loss are not panaceas for feelings of inadequacy. Overeating does appear to be a very common stress response among otherwise normal young women.

NORMAL OR NOT?

A certain degree of dieting and weight-loss behavior among teenagers can be considered normal. It is natural that young people, faced with the myriad of societal pressures to be thin, are occasionally concerned about food and weight and may watch or worry about what they eat. There is a big difference, however, between normal teenage concerns about food and/or weight and disordered eating behaviors.

(continued...)

OVERCOMING EATING DISORDERS

A teenager with the following characteristics is exhibiting normal eating behavior:
- Eats reasonable portions of foods.
- Usually eats balanced meals with a variety of foods.
- Eats the same types and amounts of food whether eating with others or alone.
- Eats enough to maintain a reasonable body weight.
- Exercises regularly for fitness.
- *Sometimes* eats as a response to stress.
- *Sometimes* diets in response to body-image concerns.

The following characteristics are signals of a possible eating disorder:
- When eating with others, eats nothing or plays with food.
- Uses purging or vomiting to get rid of food.
- Binges—eats large amounts of food within a short time.
- Plans eating binges.
- Exercises to be slim and to use up calories. May exercise excessively.
- Prefers to eat alone.
- Appears to be obsessed with thoughts of food.

Teens who exhibit any of these signs may be at risk for an eating disorder.

TREATMENT FOR EATING DISORDERS

Anorexia nervosa and bulimia are dangerous responses to body-image concerns. Appropriate eating and exercise behaviors can help many people control weight and develop a comfortable body image. Individuals with clinical eating disorders, however, need treatment that helps them develop increased self-esteem, a more accurate perception of body weight and size, and focuses on *attitudes* about food and eating rather than eating habits per se.

Eating disorders can be overcome with early detection and prompt, professional intervention. A variety of treatments are available. Depending on the severity of the disorder, hospitalization may be required. Dehydration, electrolyte imbalance, distorted thinking, heart arrhythmias and other problems associated with starvation require immediate hospitalization.

Some hospitals offer special programs for treating eating disorders. Some are inpatient in regular hospitals; others are located in psychiatric hospitals. Some hospital programs stress weight gain, others stress therapy.

(continued...)

OVERCOMING EATING DISORDERS

In addition to medical intervention to help patients regain lost weight, programs must include a combination of long-term counseling and therapeutic interventions that focus on the individual and her or his family system.

Several treatments, used alone or in combination, have been successful in the treatment of eating disorders. They include the following therapies:

- *Cognitive-behavioral therapy*—Food diaries and self-reporting of eating habits and behaviors help identify and monitor both positive and negative behaviors. Behavior modification techniques are used to reward normal eating behavior and discourage self-starvation or bingeing and purging.

- *Individual therapy*—In combination with other treatments, psychological treatment can help the individual correct perceptions of body image; decrease feelings of depression, guilt and anxiety; enhance self-esteem and assertiveness; learn stress management skills; and monitor weight.

- *Group psychotherapy* may help reduce a person's sense of isolation and secrecy. This treatment may be especially effective for bulimics. Guided by a trained professional, this type of therapy can be a useful and powerful adjunct to recovery.

- *Family therapy*—The dynamics of the family play a pivotal role in the development of eating disorders. Therefore, family members, including parents, siblings, spouses and significant others, must be involved in the treatment plan. They should be encouraged to provide a supportive recovery environment for the patient.

- *Drug therapy*—Since depression and anxiety often accompany eating disorders, medications may be prescribed as part of the treatment program. Vitamin and mineral supplements may also be prescribed.

- *Bibliotherapy*—Reading real-life accounts of other people with eating disorders may be a prescribed part of a treatment program.

- *Reality imaging*   Photographs and videotapes and computer imaging are often used to help the patient correct a distorted body image, especially when the body is emaciated but still perceived as fat.

- *Guided imagery* teaches patients to shift their focus from perceived body flaws to positive attributes.

- *Biofeedback training and relaxation techniques* may help a person overcome stress and gain more control of feelings.

(continued...)

OVERCOMING EATING DISORDERS

- *Education*—Nutritionists, registered dietitians and other diet specialists work with therapists and physicians to teach the patient appropriate healthy eating habits and educate about nutrition.
- *Hypnotherapy*—Limited success has been experienced using hypnosis as a treatment for eating disorders. Hypnosis requires the patient to relinquish control—something most eating disorder patients resist.
- *Self-help or support groups* can be used as an adjunct to primary treatment. Through sharing experiences, members give mutual emotional support, exchange information and diminish feelings of isolation. Services may include information on symptoms and treatment, lists of therapists, newsletters, book reviews and bibliographies.

FINAL EVALUATION

FINAL EVALUATION

The final evaluation is based on the game show "Jeopardy." Students use what they have learned about body image and eating disorders to provide the correct "question" when given information about terms and concepts.

GETTING STARTED

Have:

- 25 Post-it notes (1-1/2" x 2")

Make transparency of:

- Jeopardy Game Board final evaluation

SPECIAL STEPS

Place Post-its over the squares on the **Jeopardy Game Board** transparency. The answers should be covered until students choose them. Write the point value of the square on each Post-it, if time permits.

FINAL EVALUATION

Establish teams

Divide the class into 2 teams by having students count off 1-2, 1-2, or some other method. Have each team choose a captain. Flip a coin to see which team will start the game.

Explain game

Display the Jeopardy Game Board transparency, with the squares covered by Post-its. Explain the rules for the game:

- The team captain or the first member of the starting team selects a category and point value from the game board.
- The teacher will remove the Post-it to reveal the "answer."
- The team then has 30 seconds to come up with the correct response in the form of a question. Anyone from the team can respond. Team captains can monitor to be sure all team members have a chance to respond.
- If the team answers correctly, they select a new square. If they answer incorrectly, the other team has a chance to respond, and gains control of the board if correct.

(continued...)

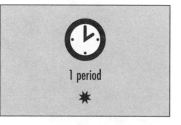

1 period

REVIEW
- Jeopardy *Key* (p. 65)

MATERIALS
- transparency of Jeopardy Game Board final evaluation
- Post-it notes

JEOPARDY GAME BOARD

FINAL EVALUATION

BODY IMAGE AND EATING DISORDERS

POINTS	TERMS (Unit 1)	CULTURE AND MEDIA (Unit 2)	EATING DISORDERS (Unit 3)	HELP FOR EATING DISORDERS (Unit 4)	POTPOURRI (All Units)
10	The way you view and believe others view your body	Means of communication that convey messages to the public	Disorder characterized by self-imposed starvation and refusal to maintain or gain weight	A course of action to stop a disease	Ability to critically interpret messages from the media
20	A measure of how you value yourself	10% or more above desirable weight	Absence or cessation of menstruation	Conforming with an accepted standard; natural	An event that sets off a cycle of strict dieting or bingeing and purging
30	Traits, including physical, mental/emotional, social and personality traits	Ideas, customs, skills and arts of a people or group	Disorder characterized by binge eating followed by purging, fasting or exercise	Anything that triggers a stress response	An image or model thought of as perfect
40	Psychological well-being; the capacity to cope with life situations	Condition in which an excessive proportion of body tissue is fat; 20% or more above desirable weight	Eating a very large amount of food at one time	Sharing sensitive or personal information with another person	Members give emotional help, share experience, exchange information; used in addition to primary treatment
50	Characteristics that provide a sense of self and others	★Double Points★ Media; family and cultural perceptions; physical characteristics; and self-esteem ★Double Points★	Attempts to rid body of food (vomiting, laxative, and/or diuretic abuse)	Like yourself as you are. Set realistic goals. Learn about nutrition and exercise. Ask for support. Seek help.	★Double Points★ 4 drugs abused by people with eating disorders ★Double Points★

© ETR Associates

Choosing Health High School

- If both teams answer incorrectly, the last team to respond correctly to a question gets control of the board.
- After all squares have been chosen, teams have a chance to wager points on the Final Jeopardy question.
- The team with the most points wins.

Play the game

Play the Jeopardy game, using the **Jeopardy Key** as a guide. Keep score for each team.

When all squares have been revealed, read the Final Jeopardy category from the **Jeopardy Key**. Allow teams to confer and wager points on the final question. When both teams have recorded their wagers, read the Final Jeopardy question and give teams time to write down their answers. Read the correct response and have teams reveal their answers and point wagers.

Total points for the teams and announce the winning team. Congratulate both teams on their knowledge and efforts.

JEOPARDY
KEY

POINTS	TERMS (Unit 1)	CULTURE AND MEDIA (Unit 2)	EATING DISORDERS (Unit 3)	HELP FOR EATING DISORDERS (Unit 4)	POTPOURRI (All Units)
10	What is body image?	What are media?	What is anorexia nervosa?	What is treatment?	What is media literacy?
20	What is self-esteem?	What is overweight?	What is amenorrhea?	What is "normal"?	What is a trigger?
30	What are personal characteristics?	What is culture?	What is bulimia?	What is a stressor?	What is ideal?
40	What is mental health?	What is obesity?	What is bingeing?	What is confiding?	What is a support group or self-help group?
50	What are social traits?	★Double Points★ What are 4 influences on body image? ★Double Points★	What is purging?	★Double Points★ What are some ways to prevent eating disorders? ★Double Points★	What are laxatives, diuretics, ipecac syrup and diet pills?

FINAL JEOPARDY

Category: Eating disorders

Clue: 5 factors that influence eating disorder behaviors

Response: What are psychological factors, family problems, lifestyle factors, biological factors and nutrition?

© ETR Associates

APPENDIXES

Why Comprehensive School Health?

Components of a
Comprehensive Health Program

The Teacher's Role

Teaching Strategies

Glossary

References

Why Comprehensive School Health?

The quality of life we ultimately achieve is determined in large part by the health decisions we make, the subsequent behaviors we adopt, and the public policies that promote and support the establishment of healthy behaviors.

A healthy student is capable of growing and learning; of producing new knowledge and ideas; of sharing, interacting and living peacefully with others in a complex and changing society. Fostering healthy children is the shared responsibility of families, communities and schools.

Health behaviors, the most important predictors of current and future health status, are influenced by a variety of factors. Factors that lead to and support the establishment of healthy behaviors include:

- awareness and knowledge of health issues
- the skills necessary to practice healthy behaviors
- opportunities to practice healthy behaviors
- support and reinforcement for the practice of healthy behaviors

The perception that a particular healthy behavior is worthwhile often results in young people becoming advocates, encouraging others to adopt the healthy behavior. When these young advocates exert pressure on peers to adopt healthy behaviors, a healthy social norm is established (e.g., tobacco use is unacceptable in this school).

Because health behaviors are learned, they can be shaped and changed. Partnerships between family members, community leaders, teachers and school leaders are a vital key to the initial development and maintenance of children's healthy behaviors and can also play a role in the modification of unhealthy behaviors. Schools, perhaps more than any other single agency in our society, have the opportunity to influence factors that shape the future health and productivity of Americans.

When young people receive reinforcement for the practice of a healthy behavior, they feel good about the healthy behavior. Reinforcement and the subsequent good feeling increase the likelihood that an individual will continue to practice a behavior and thereby establish a positive health habit. The good feeling and the experience of success motivate young people to place a high value on the behavior (e.g., being a nonsmoker is good).

From *Step by Step to Comprehensive School Health,* W. M. Kane (Santa Cruz, CA: ETR Associates, 1992).

COMPONENTS OF A COMPREHENSIVE HEALTH PROGRAM

The school's role in fostering the development of healthy students involves more than providing classes in health. There are 8 components of a comprehensive health education program:

- **School Health Instruction**—Instruction is the in-class aspect of the program. As in other subject areas, a scope of content defines the field. Application of classroom instruction to real life situations is critical.

- **Healthy School Environment**—The school environment includes both the physical and psychological surroundings of students, faculty and staff. The physical environment should be free of hazards; the psychological environment should foster healthy development.

- **School Health Services**—School health services offer a variety of activities that address the health status of students and staff.

- **Physical Education and Fitness**—Participation in physical education and fitness activities promotes healthy development. Students need information about how and why to be active and encouragement to develop skills that will contribute to fitness throughout their lives.

- **School Nutrition and Food Services**—The school's nutritional program provides an excellent opportunity to model healthy behaviors. Schools that provide healthy food choices and discourage availability of unhealthy foods send a clear message to students about the importance of good nutrition.

- **School-Based Counseling and Personal Support**—School counseling and support services play an important role in responding to special needs and providing personal support for individual students, teachers and staff. These services can also provide programs that promote schoolwide mental, emotional and social well-being.

- **Schoolsite Health Promotion**—Health promotion is a combination of educational, organizational and environmental activities designed to encourage students and staff to adopt healthier lifestyles and become better consumers of health care services. It views the school and its activities as a total environment.

- **School, Family and Community Health Promotion Partnerships**— Partnerships that unite schools, families and communities can address communitywide issues. These collaborative partnerships are the cornerstone of health promotion and disease prevention.

THE TEACHER'S ROLE

The teacher plays a critical role in meeting the challenge to empower students with the knowledge, skills and ability to make healthy behavior choices throughout their lives.

Instruction

Teachers need to provide students with learning opportunities that go beyond knowledge. Instruction must include the chance to practice skills that will help students make healthy decisions.

Involve Families and Communities

The issues in health are real-life issues, issues that families and communities deal with daily. Students need to see the relationship of what they learn at school to what occurs in their homes and their communities.

Model Healthy Behavior

Teachers educate students by their actions too. Students watch the way teachers manage health issues in their own lives. Teachers need to ask themselves if they are modeling the health behaviors they want students to adopt.

Maintain a Healthy Environment

The classroom environment has both physical and emotional aspects. It is the teacher's role to maintain a safe physical environment. It is also critical to provide an environment that is sensitive, respectful and developmentally appropriate.

Establish Groundrules

It is very important to establish classroom groundrules before discussing sensitive topics or issues. Setting and consistently enforcing groundrules establishes an atmosphere of respect, in which students can share and explore their personal thoughts, feelings, opinions and values.

Refer Students to Appropriate Services

Teachers may be the first to notice illness, learning disorders or emotional distress in students. The role of the teacher is one of referral. Most districts have guidelines for teachers to follow.

Legal Compliance

Teachers must make every effort to communicate to parents and other family members about the nature of the curriculum. Instruction about certain topics, such as sexuality, HIV or drug use, often must follow notification guidelines regulated by state law. Most states also require teachers to report any suspected cases of child abuse or neglect.

TEACHING STRATEGIES

The resource books incorporate a variety of instructional strategies. This variety is essential in addressing the needs of different kinds of learners. Different strategies are grouped according to their general education purpose. When sequenced, these strategies are designed to help students acquire the knowledge and skills they need to choose healthy behavior. Strategies are identified with each activity. Some strategies are traditional, while others are more interactive, encouraging students to help each other learn.

The strategies are divided into 4 categories according to their general purpose:

- providing key information
- encouraging creative expression
- sharing thoughts, feelings and opinions
- developing critical thinking

The following list details strategies in each category.

Providing Key Information

Information provides the foundation for learning. Before students can move to higher-level thinking, they need to have information about a topic. In lieu of a textbook, this series uses a variety of strategies to provide students the information they need to take actions for their health.

Anonymous Question Box

An anonymous question box provides the opportunity for all students to get answers to questions they might be hesitant to ask in class. It also gives teachers time to think about answers to difficult questions or to look for more information.

Questions should be reviewed and responded to regularly, and all questions placed in the box should be taken seriously. If you don't know the answer to a question, research it and report back to students.

You may feel that some questions would be better answered privately. Offer students the option of signing their questions if they want a private, written answer. Any questions not answered in class can then be answered privately.

Current Events

Analyzing local, state, national and international current events helps students relate classroom discussion to everyday life. It also helps students understand how local, national and global events and policies affect health status. Resources for current events include newspapers, magazines and other periodicals, radio and television programs and news.

Demonstrations and Experiments

Teachers, guest speakers or students can use demonstrations and experiments to show how something works or why something is important. These activities also provide a way to show the correct process for doing something, such as a first-aid procedure.

Demonstrations and experiments should be carefully planned and conducted. They often involve the use of supporting materials.

Games and Puzzles

Games and puzzles can be used to provide a different environment in which learning can take place. They are frequently amusing and sometimes competitive.

Many types of games and puzzles can be adapted to present and review health concepts. It may be a simple question-and-answer game or an adaptation of games such as Bingo, Concentration or Jeopardy. Puzzles include crosswords and word searches.

A game is played according to a specific set of rules. Game rules should be clear and simple. Using groups of students in teams rather than individual contestants helps involve the entire class.

Guest Speakers

Guest speakers can be recruited from students' families, the school and the community. They provide a valuable link between the classroom and the "real world."

Speakers should be screened before being invited to present to the class. They should have some awareness of the level of student knowledge and should be given direction for the content and focus of the presentation.

Interviewing

Students can interview experts and others about a specific topic either inside or outside of class. Invite experts, family members and others to visit class, or ask students to interview others (family members or friends) outside of class.

Advance preparation for an organized interview session increases the learning potential. A brainstorming session before the interview allows students to develop questions to ask during the interview.

TEACHING STRATEGIES

Oral Presentations

Individual students or groups or panels of students can present information orally to the rest of the class. Such presentations may sometimes involve the use of charts or posters to augment the presentation.

Students enjoy learning and hearing from each other, and the experience stimulates positive interaction. It also helps build students' communication skills.

Encouraging Creative Expression

Student creativity should be encouraged and challenged. Creative expression provides the opportunity to integrate language arts, fine arts and personal experience into a lesson. It also helps meet the diverse needs of students with different learning styles.

Artistic Expression or Creative Writing

Students may be offered a choice of expressing themselves in art or through writing. They may write short stories, poems or letters, or create pictures or collages about topics they are studying. Such a choice accommodates the differing needs and talents of students.

This technique can be used as a follow-up to most lessons. Completed work should be displayed in the classroom, at school or in the community.

Dramatic Presentations

Dramatic presentations may take the form of skits or mock news, radio or television shows. They can be presented to the class or to larger groups in the school or community. When equipment is available, videotapes of these presentations provide an opportunity to present students' work to other classes in the school and other groups in the community.

Such presentations are highly motivating activities, because they actively involve students in learning desired concepts. They also allow students to practice new behaviors in a safe setting and help them personalize information presented in class.

Roleplays

Acting out difficult situations provides students practice in new behaviors in a safe setting. Sometimes students are given a part to play, and other times they are given an idea and asked to improvise. Students need time to decide the central action of the situation and how they will resolve it before they make their presentation. Such activities are highly motivating because they actively involve students in learning desired concepts or practicing certain behaviors.

Sharing Thoughts, Feelings and Opinions

In the sensitive areas of health education, students may have a variety of opinions and feelings. Providing a safe atmosphere in which to discuss opinions and feelings encourages students to share their ideas and listen and learn from others. Such discussion also provides an opportunity to clarify misinformation and correct misconceptions.

Brainstorming

Brainstorming is used to stimulate discussion of an issue or topic. It can be done with the whole class or in smaller groups. It can be used both to gather information and to share thoughts and opinions.

All statements should be accepted without comment or judgment from the teacher or other students. Ideas can be listed on the board, on butcher paper or newsprint or on a transparency. Brainstorming should continue until all ideas have been exhausted or a predetermined time limit has been reached.

Class Discussion

A class discussion led by the teacher or by students is a valuable educational strategy. It can be used to initiate, amplify or summarize a lesson. Such discussions also provide a way to share ideas, opinions and concerns that may have been generated in small group work.

Clustering

Clustering is a simple visual technique that involves diagraming ideas around a main topic. The main topic is written on the board and circled. Other related ideas are then attached to the central idea or to each other with connecting lines.

Clustering can be used as an adjunct to brainstorming. Because there is no predetermined number of secondary ideas, clustering can accommodate all brainstorming ideas.

Continuum Voting

Continuum voting is a stimulating discussion technique. Students express the extent to which they agree or disagree with a statement read by the teacher. The classroom

TEACHING STRATEGIES

should be prepared for this activity with a sign that says "Agree" on one wall and a sign that says "Disagree" on the opposite wall. There should be room for students to move freely between the 2 signs.

As the teacher reads a statement, students move to a point between the signs that reflects their thoughts or feelings. The closer to the "Agree" sign they stand, the stronger their agreement. The closer to the "Disagree" sign they stand, the stronger their disagreement. A position in the center between the signs indicates a neutral stance.

Dyad Discussion

Working in pairs allows students to provide encouragement and support to each other. Students who may feel uncomfortable sharing in the full class may be more willing to share their thoughts and feelings with 1 other person. Depending on the task, dyads may be temporary, or students may meet regularly with a partner and work together to achieve their goals.

Forced Field Analysis

This strategy is used to discuss an issue that is open to debate. Students analyze a situation likely to be approved by some students and opposed by others. For example, if the subject of discussion was the American diet, some students might support the notion that Americans consume healthy foods because of the wide variety of foods available. Other students might express concern about the amount of foods that are high in sodium, fat and sugar.

Questioning skills are critical to the success of this technique. A good way to open such a discussion is to ask students, "What questions should you ask to determine if you support or oppose this idea?" The pros and cons of students' analysis can be charted on the board or on a transparency.

Journal Writing

Journal writing affords the opportunity for thinking and writing. Expressive writing requires that students become actively involved in the learning process. However, writing may become a less effective tool for learning if students must worry about spelling and punctuation. Students should be encouraged to write freely in their journals, without fear of evaluation.

Panel Discussion

Panel discussions provide an opportunity to discuss different points of view about a health topic, problem or issue. Students can research and develop supporting arguments for different sides. Such research and discussion enhances understanding of content.

Panel members may include experts from the community as well as students. Panel discussions are usually directed by a moderator and may be followed by a question and answer period.

Self-Assessment

Personal inventories provide a tool for self-assessment. Providing privacy around personal assessments allows students to be honest in their responses. Volunteers can share answers or the questions can be discussed in general, but no students should have to share answers they would prefer to keep private. Students can use the information to set personal goals for changing behaviors.

Small Groups

Students working together can help stimulate each other's creativity. Small group activities are cooperative, but have less formal structure than cooperative learning groups. These activities encourage collective thinking and provide opportunities for students to work with others and increase social skills.

Surveys and Inventories

Surveys and inventories can be used to assess knowledge, attitudes, beliefs and practices. These instruments can be used to gather knowledge about a variety of groups, including students, parents and other family members, and teachers.

Students can use surveys others have designed or design their own. When computers are available, students can use them to summarize their information, create graphs and prepare presentations of the data.

Developing Critical Thinking

Critical thinking skills help students analyze health topics and issues. These activities require that students learn to gather information, consider the consequences of actions and behaviors and make responsible decisions. They challenge students to perform higher-level thinking and clearly communicate their ideas.

Case Studies

Case studies provide written histories of a problem or situation. Students can read, discuss and analyze these situations. This strategy encourages student involvement and helps students personalize the health-related concepts presented in class.

TEACHING STRATEGIES

Cooperative Learning Groups

Cooperative learning is an effective teaching strategy that has been shown to have a positive effect on students' achievement and interpersonal skills. Students can work in small groups to disseminate and share information, analyze ideas or solve problems. The size of the group depends on the nature of the lesson and the make-up of the class. Groups work best with from 2–6 members.

Group structure will affect the success of the lessons. Groups can be formed by student choice, random selection, or a more formal, teacher-influenced process. Groups seem to function best when they represent the variety and balance found in the classroom. Groups also work better when each student has a responsibility within the group (reader, recorder, timer, reporter, etc.).

While groups are working on their tasks, the teacher should move from group to group, answering questions and dealing with any problems that arise. At the conclusion of the group process, some closure should take place.

Debates

Students can debate the pros and cons of many issues relating to health. Suggesting that students defend an opposing point of view provides an additional learning experience.

During a debate, each side has the opportunity to present their arguments and to refute each others' arguments. After the debate, class members can choose the side with which they agree.

Factual Writing

Once students have been presented with information about a topic, a variety of writing assignments can challenge them to clarify and express their ideas and opinions. Position papers, letters to the editor, proposals and public service announcements provide a forum in which students can express their opinions, supporting them with facts, figures and reasons.

Media Analysis

Students can analyze materials from a variety of media, including printed matter, music, TV programs, movies, video games and advertisements, to identify health-related messages. Such analysis might include identifying the purpose of the piece, the target audience, underlying messages, motivations and stereotypes.

TEACHING STRATEGIES

Personal Contracts

Personal contracts, individual commitments to changing behavior, can help students make positive changes in their health-related behaviors. The wording of a personal contract may include the behavior to be changed, a plan for changing the behavior and the identification of possible problems and support systems.

However, personal contracts should be used with caution. Behavior change may be difficult, especially in the short term. Students should be encouraged to make personal contracts around goals they are likely to meet.

Research

Research requires students to seek information to complete a task. Students may be given prepared materials that they must use to complete an assignment, or they may have to locate resources and gather information on their own. As part of this strategy, students must compile and organize the information they collect.

GLOSSARY

A

addiction—Physical or psychological condition of dependence on a drug or habit.

additive—A substance that has been added to food to produce a desired effect, such as a preservative.

advertising—Public announcements of the qualities or advantages of a product or service.

alternatives—Choices of things to do.

amenorrhea—The absence or cessation of menstruation.

amino acids—Chemicals that are the building blocks of proteins.

anemia—A condition in which blood lacks red blood cells or the cells are deficient in hemoglobin.

anorexia nervosa—An eating disorder characterized by self-starvation and refusal to maintain a minimally normal body weight.

atherosclerosis—A disease in which the arteries become clogged with fats and other substances that form plaques.

B

balance—The proportion of various elements or foods.

binge—Eating an extraordinarily large amount of food at one time.

body—The physical structure and substance of a human being.

body composition—The proportion of body muscle to body fat.

body image—The way an individual views and believes others view his or her body.

bulimia—An eating disorder characterized by repeated episodes of binge eating followed by purging behaviors such as self-induced vomiting, misuse of laxatives and diuretics, fasting and excessive exercising.

C

calcium—A mineral needed for growth and maintenance of strong bones and teeth.

calorie—A unit for measuring heat energy and the energy value of foods.

carbohydrate—A nutrient composed of carbon, hydrogen and oxygen; the body's preferred form of energy.

cathartic—Term often used interchangeably with laxative; stronger, faster-acting or higher-dose laxative.

cognitive-behavioral therapy—Therapy that uses self-assessment and behavior modification techniques to help change patterns of behavior.

confide—To share sensitive or personal information with another person.

culture—Ideas, customs, skills and arts of a people or group.

GLOSSARY

D

dehydrated—Dry; lacking water in the body tissues.

dehydration—Loss of water from the body tissues.

dietary fiber—Plant material in food; may be soluble or insoluble.

dieting—Limiting food and drink to produce weight loss.

diuretic—A drug that helps relieve the body of excess water by increasing the excretion of urine.

drug—A chemical substance that has a direct effect on the structure or function of the body; any substance that causes a physical or mental change in the body.

dysmorphophobia—An obsession in which a person fixates on a particular body flaw, blowing it out of proportion.

E

eating disorder—A serious and health-threatening upset in patterns of food consumption.

electrolytes—Compounds that partially dissociate in water to form ions.

electronic media—Media that require electricity to operate and communicate messages.

empty calorie food—Foods high in calories but lacking in nutrient value (e.g., soft drinks, cookies, cakes, candy and many snack foods).

energy—A measure of the ability to do work.

esophagitis—Inflammation or irritation of the esophagus.

esophagus—The tube that links the throat and the stomach.

essential—Required, as nutrients required by the body for normal function.

F

fast—To go without food for a designated period of time.

fat—A nutrient that is the body's second major source of energy and the preferred means of storing energy.

food—Nourishment; any substance taken into the body to keep it alive.

H

health—The general condition of the body.

I

ideal—An image or model that is thought of as perfect.

image—An imitation, representation or impression of a person or thing; a likeness.

influence—The ability of a person or thing to affect others.

GLOSSARY

iron—A mineral used by the body to make *hemoglobin*, the part of the blood that moves oxygen from the lungs to the body tissue.

L

laxative—Substance that loosens the bowels and relieves constipation.

laxative abuse—Use of laxatives for the purpose of weight control.

M

media—Means of communication, such as newspapers, radio and TV, that provide information and convey messages to the public; includes print (newspapers, billboards, magazines, mail), electronic (telephone, computer on-line services), broadcast (television, radio), and the arts.

media literacy—The ability to read, critically analyze, evaluate and produce communications in a variety of media.

mental/emotional traits—Characteristics that relate to feelings, perceptions, experiences, personal relationships, inner conflicts, sexuality, impulses, moodiness and coping mechanisms.

mental health—Psychological well-being; the capacity to cope with life situations, grow emotionally through them, develop to the fullest potential and grow in awareness and consciousness.

metabolism—Continuous chemical and physical processes in the body.

metabolize—To change by a chemical process.

mineral—An inorganic substance required by the body for metabolism.

moderation—The avoidance of extremes; freedom from excess; restraint.

mood—A person's sustained and predominant internal emotional experience (e.g., depression, euphoria).

N

normal—Conforming with an accepted standard; natural; common, usual or typical.

nutrient—A chemical substance found in food that the body needs for proper growth and function.

nutrient density—A measure of the nutritional value of foods, based on the relationship of nutritional value to caloric value.

nutrition—The science of food and how it is used in the body.

O

obesity—A condition in which an excessive proportion of body tissue is fat; judged by a criterion of being 20% or more above desirable weight.

over-the-counter medication—Medication that can be purchased without a doctor's prescription.

overweight—A condition of being 10% or more above desirable weight. Overweight people are not necessarily obese.

P

perfect—Without flaw.

perfectionism—An obsessive striving for perfection.

personal characteristics—Those traits or characteristics that make up an individual, including physical, mental/emotional, social and personality traits.

personality—Unique constellation of emotions, thoughts and behaviors that determine who a person is and how each person functions and adapts to life.

personality traits—Attitudes, habits, emotions and thoughts that produce a characteristic way of behaving.

physical traits—Characteristics that relate to the body and appearance. During adolescence, changes in physical characteristics include growth spurts and appearance of secondary sex characteristics.

potassium—A mineral that helps stimulate the nerves that help muscles contract; needed for normal growth.

prescription—A doctor's written direction for the preparation and use of a medicine.

prescription drug—Controlled substance that must be used under the direction of a physician.

prevention—Hindering or stopping something from happening or existing.

privacy—One's private life; those things kept secret or closely guarded.

psychological—Having to do with the mind, both normal and abnormal states.

purgative—Term often used interchangeably with *laxative*; stronger, faster-acting or higher-dose laxative.

purging—Attempts to rid the body of food, including self-induced vomiting, or diuretic or laxative abuse.

R

risk—The likelihood of injury, damage or other negative consequences following an action.

ritual—An established form or ceremony.

GLOSSARY

S

self-concept—Refers to what the individual thinks, feels and believes about the self; a conscious set of beliefs about oneself that influence behavior.

self-esteem—Measure of how much a person values himself or herself.

social traits—Characteristics that provide a sense of self and others. Goal setting, peer group affiliation, building relationships and practicing interpersonal skills are social characteristics.

starvation—Dying or death from lack of food.

stress—The feeling of being under pressure; bodily wear and tear caused by physical or psychological arousal.

stressor—Anything that triggers a stress response (e.g., external events, internal reactions).

support group—A group of people with similar concerns or behaviors who meet regularly to offer each other emotional support and to exchange information.

survival—The act of staying alive.

symptoms—Subjective evidence of disease; indications of the presence of a bodily disorder.

T

therapy—The treatment of a physical or mental disorder by medical or psychological means.

trachea—Windpipe; the tube that connects the throat and the lungs.

treatment—The techniques or actions applied in a certain situation, such as medically caring for a patient; a course of action to stop a disease.

trigger—An event or action that sets off a certain behavior cycle.

V

vitamin—An organic compound found in foods that is essential to normal metabolism and helps regulate body processes.

vomit—To eject the contents of the stomach through the mouth; throw up.

Y

yo-yo syndrome—The process of losing and regaining weight in an ongoing cycle.

REFERENCES

Biener, L., and A. Heaton. 1995. Women dieters of normal weight: Their motives, goals and risks. *American Journal of Public Health* 85 (5): 714-717.

Brodie, D. A., K. Bagley and P. D. Slade. 1994. Body-image perception in pre- and postadolescent females. *Perceptual and Motor Skills* 78:147-154.

Brownell, K. D., and T. A. Wadden. 1986. Behavior therapy for obesity: Modern approaches and better results. In *Handbook of eating disorders: Physiology; psychology; and treatment of obesity, anorexia, and bulimia,* ed. K. D. Brownell and J. P. Foreyt, 180-187. New York: Basic Books.

Brownell, K. D., and T. A. Wadden. 1992. Etiology and treatment of obesity: Understanding a serious prevalent and refractory disorder. *Journal of Consulting and Clinical Psychology* 60 (4): 505-517

Bruch, H. 1975. Emotional aspects of obesity in children. *Pediatric Annals* 4:91.

California Task Force to Promote Self-Esteem and Personal and Social Responsibility. 1990. *Toward a state of esteem.* Sacramento: California State Department of Education.

Cavior, N., and D. A. Lombardi. 1973. Developmental aspects of judgment of physical attractiveness in children. *Developmental Psychology* 8:67-71.

Council on Scientific Affairs. 1988. Treatment of obesity in adults. *Journal of the American Medical Association* 260:2547-2551.

Crisp, A. H. 1988. Some possible approaches to prevention of eating and body weight/shape disorders, with particular reference to anorexia nervosa. *International Journal of Eating Disorders* 7:1-17.

Diagnostic and statistical manual of mental disorders (DSM-IV). 4th ed. 1994. Washington, DC: American Psychiatric Association.

Evans, N., E. Gilpin, A. J. Farkas, E. Shenassa and J. P. Pierce. 1995. Adolescents' perceptions of their peers' health norms. *American Journal of Public Health* 85 (8): 1064-1069.

Fetro, J. V. 1992. *Personal and social skills: Understanding and integrating competencies across health content.* Santa Cruz, CA: ETR Associates.

Foreyt, J. P., and G. K. Goodrick. 1994. What can we do about obesity in the U.S.? *Healthy Weight Journal* 8 (3): 50.

French, S. A., M. Story, B. Downes, M. D. Resnick and R. W. Blum. 1995. Frequent dieting among adolescents: Psychosocial and health behavior correlates. *American Journal of Public Health* 85 (5): 695-701.

Gralen, S. J., M. P. Levine, L. Smolak and S. K. Murnen. 1990. Dieting and disordered eating during early and middle adolescence: Do the influences remain the same? *International Journal of Eating Disorders* 9 (5): 501-512.

REFERENCES

Grant, C. L., and I. R. Fodor. 1986. Adolescent attitudes toward body image and anorexic behavior. *Adolescence* 21:269-281.

Hammer, L. D. 1992. The development of eating behavior in childhood. *Pediatric Clinics of North America* 39:279-304.

Hellmich, N. 1995. Looking thin and fit weighs on more women. *USA Today.* 25 September.

Hellmich, N. 1995. Twice as many kids overweight. *USA Today.* 3 October.

Herzog, D., and P. Copeland. 1985. Eating disorders. *New England Journal of Medicine* 313:295-303.

Heunemann, R. L., L. R. Shapiro, M. C. Hampton and B. W. Mitchell. 1966. A longitudinal study of gross body composition and body conformation and their association with food and activity in a teenage population. *American Journal of Clinical Nutrition* 18:325-338.

Kann, L., C. W. Warren, W. A. Harris, J. L. Collins, K. A. Douglas, M. E. Collins, B. I. Williams, J. G. Ross and L. J. Kolbe. 1995. Youth risk behavior surveillance—United States, 1993. In CDC Surveillance Summaries, *Morbidity and Mortality Weekly Report* 44 (SS-1): 1-56.

Lerner, R. M., and J. Jovanovic. 1990. *The role of body image in psychosocial development across the lifespan: A developmental contextual perspective.* New York: Guilford Press.

Lloyd-Kolkin, D., and K. R. Tyner. 1991. *Media and you.* San Francisco: Strategies for Media Literacy.

McGinnis, M. J., and W. H. Foege. 1993. Actual causes of death in the United States. *Journal of the American Medical Association* 270 (18): 2207-2212.

Mitchell, J., and E. Eckert. 1987. Scope and significance of eating disorders. *Journal of Consulting Clinical Psychologist* 55:628-634.

Morris, A., T. Cooper and P. Cooper. 1989. The changing shape of female fashion models. *International Journal of Eating Disorders* 8 (5): 593-596.

National Association of Anorexia Nervosa and Associated Disorders (ANAD). n.d. *Media Page.* Highland Park, IL.

Papazian, R. 1991. Never say diet. *FDA Consumer.* DHHS Publication No. (FDA) 92-1188. Washington, DC: U.S. Government Printing Office.

Patton, G. C., E. Johnson-Sabine, K. Woods, A. H. Mann and A. Wakeling. 1990. Abnormal eating attitudes in London school girls: outcome at twelve month follow-up. *Psychological Medicine* 20:383-394.

Paxton, S. J., E. H. Wertheim, K. Gibbons, G. I. Szmukler, L. Hillier and J. L. Petrovich. 1991. Body image satisfaction, dieting beliefs and weight loss behaviors in adolescent girls and boys. *Journal of Youth and Adolescence* 20:361-379.

REFERENCES

Paxton, S. J. 1993. A prevention program for disturbed eating and body dissatisfaction in adolescent girls: A 1 year follow-up. *Health Education Research Theory and Practice,* 8 (1): 43-51.

Rosen, J. C., and J. Gross. 1987. Prevalence of weight reducing and weight gaining in adolescent girls and boys. *Health Psychology* 6:131-147.

Rosen, J. C., J. Gross and L. Vara. 1987. Psychological adjustments of adolescents attempting to lose or gain weight. *Journal of Consulting and Clinical Psychology* 55:742-747.

Shisslak, C. M., M. Crago, M. E. Neal and B. Swain. 1987. Primary prevention of eating disorders. *Journal of Consulting and Clinical Psychology* 55:660-667.

Silverstein, B., L. Perdue, B. Peterson and E. Kelly. 1986. The role of the mass media in promoting a thin standard of bodily attractiveness for women. *Sex Roles* 14 (9/10): 519-532.

Social stigma of overweight hits hard. 1994. *Healthy Weight Journal* 8 (3): 46.

Staffieri, J. R. 1967. A study of social stereotype of body image in children. *Journal of Personality and Social Psychology* 7:101-104.

Stang, L., and K. R. Miner. 1994. *Nutrition and body image: Health facts.* Santa Cruz, CA: ETR Associates.

Storm, P. 1987. *Functions of dress: Culture and the individual.* Englewood Cliffs, NJ: Prentice-Hall Publishing.

Stunkard, A. J., and T. A. Wadden. 1992. Psychological aspects of severe obesity. *American Journal of Clinical Nutrition* 55 (Suppl.): 524S-532S.

Stunkard, A. J. 1993. *Obesity.* New York: Raven Press.

Thoman, E. 1993. Media literacy: Educating for today—and tomorrow. *Curriculum/Technology Quarterly* (Spring):1.

Trowbridge, F., and B. Collins. 1993. Measuring dietary behaviors among adolescents. *Public Health Reports* 108 (Suppl. 1): 37-41.

Wadden, T. A., and A. J. Stunkard. 1985. Social and psychological consequences of obesity. *Annals of Internal Medicine* 103:1062-1067.

Wertheim, E. H., S. J. Paxton, D. Maude, G. I. Szmukler, K. Gibbons and L. Hiller. 1992. Psychosocial predictors of weight loss behaviors and binge eating in adolescent girls and boys. *International Journal of Eating Disorders* 12 (2): 151-160.

Wiseman, C. V., J. J. Gray, J. E. Mosimann and A. H. Ahrens. 1992. Cultural expectations of thinness in women: An update. *International Journal of Eating Disorders* 11 (1): 85-89.

Wolf, N. 1991. *The beauty myth: How images of beauty are used against women.* New York: William Morrow.

CONTENTS

WHAT'S PERFECT?

Name _____ Date _____ Period _____

DIRECTIONS → In Part 1, write a short paragraph about your idea of a "perfect" body. If you are a male, write about a perfect male body. If you are a female, write about a perfect female body. Keep your ideas to yourself. Complete Part 2 after your class discussion.

PART 1

My opinion of a "perfect" body is...

PART 2

Some of the things that influence this view of "perfect" are...

© ETR Associates

Choosing Health High School

LOOKING AT MYSELF

Name _____ Date _____ Period _____

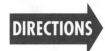 **DIRECTIONS** Using the following scale, place the number that describes your feeling about each body part or other characteristic next to that part in the diagram.

SCALE:

1 = I have strong negative feelings about this and wish I could change it.

2 = I don't like this, but I can live with it.

3 = I have no particular feelings about this.

4 = I am satisfied with this.

5 = I consider myself fortunate in this.

BODY:

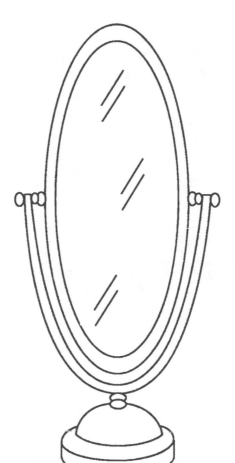

_____ 1. hair
_____ 2. facial complexion
_____ 3. appetite
_____ 4. hands
_____ 5. distribution of body hair
_____ 6. nose
_____ 7. fingers
_____ 8. wrists
_____ 9. waist
_____ 10. energy level
_____ 11. back
_____ 12. ears
_____ 13. chin
_____ 14. muscle tone
_____ 15. ankles
_____ 16. neck
_____ 17. head shape
_____ 18. body build
_____ 19. profile
_____ 20. height

_____ 21. weight
_____ 22. age
_____ 23. shoulder width
_____ 24. arms
_____ 25. chest
_____ 26. eyes
_____ 27. digestion
_____ 28. hips
_____ 29. lips
_____ 30. legs
_____ 31. teeth
_____ 32. forehead
_____ 33. feet
_____ 34. voice
_____ 35. health
_____ 36. knees
_____ 37. posture
_____ 38. face
_____ 39. fingernails
_____ 40. eyelashes

Scoring: Add up all the point values you assigned to the characteristics and divide the total by 40. Your score should fall between 1 and 5.

A score closer to 5 indicates you are very comfortable with your body image. A score closer to 1 indicates that you are very uncomfortable. You may need to think about changing your attitude to improve your self-esteem about your body image. You may also want to consider healthful ways to change your appearance.

© ETR Associates

Choosing Health High School

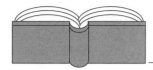

SURVIVAL NOTES

STUDENT READING

Do:

- Accept that bodies come in a variety of shapes and sizes. This makes life interesting.

- Remember that you can be your worst critic. Others may find you really attractive.

- Expect normal weekly and monthly changes in weight and shape.

- Explore your internal self—emotionally, spiritually and as a growing, changing human being.

- Explore all the things you have to offer others—caring, enthusiasm, information, companionship, love and honesty.

- Decide how you wish to spend your energy—pursuing the perfect image or enjoying family, friends and school.

- Be aware of your own prejudices about weight and body size. Explore how those feelings may affect your self-esteem.

Don't:

- Don't let your body define who or what you are. You are much more than just a body.

- Don't let obsession with your body keep you from getting close to others or doing things you want to do.

- Don't judge others on the basis of appearance, body size or shape.

- Don't forget that society changes its idea of beauty over the years.

- Don't believe that all thin people are happy with themselves.

- Don't forget that you are not alone in your pursuit of self-acceptance. It is a lifelong process that many people struggle with.

- Don't be afraid to enjoy and appreciate your body.

© ETR Associates

CHANGES

Name _____ Date _____ Period _____

DIRECTIONS ➤ Look over your answers on the **Looking at Myself** activity sheet. Choose the body areas that you marked with a 1 or 2. List those areas in the columns below as something that can be changed or something that cannot be changed. After you make these lists, answer the questions.

THINGS I *CAN* CHANGE

_____

_____

_____

_____

_____

_____

THINGS I *CANNOT* CHANGE

_____

_____

_____

_____

_____

_____

1. Choose 1 of the things you *can* change: _____

Describe what change you *can* make: _____

How can you make this change?

2. Choose 1 of the things you *cannot* change: _____

How can you work at accepting this?

© ETR Associates

BODY IMAGE PRESSURES

STUDENT READING

From early childhood, our society teaches us that appearance is very important. Feeling attractive is an essential part of self-worth. Children quickly learn that others will judge them by how they look. Success seems to be promised to those whose looks match a certain ideal.

For women, this ideal is a tall, thin, young, well-proportioned body. The male ideal is also tall, with an athletic-looking body, well-defined muscles and no evident fat. Both male and female ideals have flawless complexions and beautiful teeth. Television, movies, magazines, newspapers and billboards show us models with these features.

Most of us will never look like this. But the message we get is that we can meet this ideal if we try hard enough. When we believe this message, we can become very unhappy. We may spend many hours and a lot of money trying to change our appearance.

When we fail to achieve these impossible standards, we may feel incompetent, have low self-esteem and be depressed. Many researchers believe that eating disorders, such as anorexia nervosa and bulimia, can result from attempts to attain society's "ideal" body.

These eating disorders can be a problem both for males and females. Although more women than men have an eating disorder, at least 1 of every 10 individuals with an eating disorder is male, usually between the ages of 13 and 30.

Men and women need to develop personal skills that help them feel good about themselves. They need to recognize that dieting, exercise and dressing a certain way are not keys to success. Many messages about body image suggest that to be successful, appearance is as important as ability. According to these messages, it is not enough to simply be good at what you do, you have to look a certain way as well.

Once we understand these body image messages and the effect they can have on our self-esteem, we can develop the skills to deal with them.

© ETR Associates

CULTURAL CONNECTIONS

Name _____ Date _____ Period _____

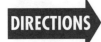 **DIRECTIONS** Write the names of the cultures that influence you in the circles. Put the culture that has the most influence in the center circle. Use the overlapping circles to identify other cultures that influence you.

Then, in each circle, write a brief description of what you believe the perception of body image held by that culture is, for both males and females.

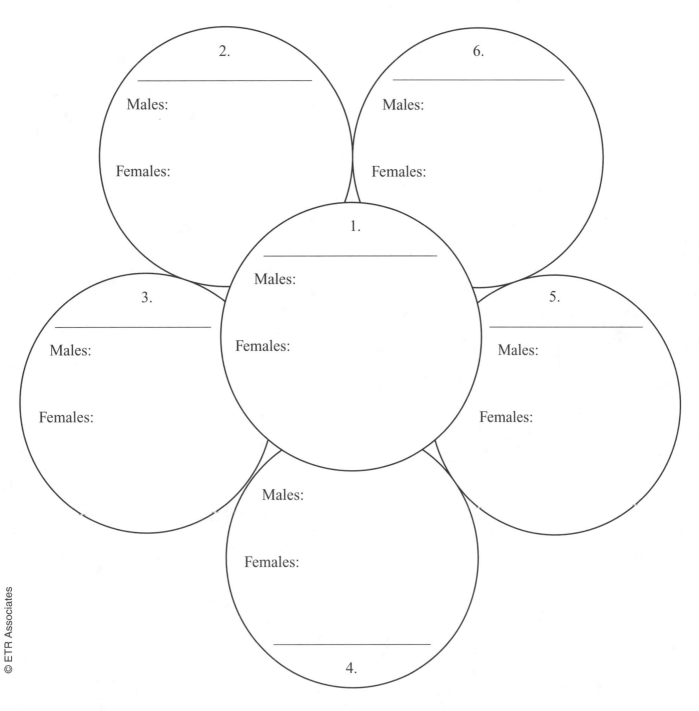

2.
_____
Males:

Females:

6.
_____
Males:

Females:

1.
_____
Males:

Females:

3.
_____
Males:

Females:

5.
_____
Males:

Females:

Males:

Females:

_____
4.

© ETR Associates

MEDIA MESSAGES

Name _____ Date _____ Period _____

DIRECTIONS ➤ Answer the questions about the advertisement you have. Use steps 1–4 in the *Scoring and Interpretation* section to analyze the results.

What is the name of the advertised product? _____

What kind of product is it? (Circle or fill in the blank.)

Diet (weight control)   Alcoholic beverage (beer, wine, liquor)
Clothing
Tobacco   Other _____

Rate the advertisement on each of the following factors, using this scale:

5 = Strongly Agree   **2** = Disagree
4 = Agree   **1** = Strongly Disagree
3 = Undecided   **0** = Not Applicable (no body-image messages included)

Circle 1 choice for each statement.

Generally, the advertisement: Score

Statement	Scale	Score
1. Suggests that use of the product will produce a positive body image.	5 4 3 2 1 0	_____
2. Shows a socially negative body image.	5 4 3 2 1 0	_____
3. Suggests the product is a solution for boredom.	5 4 3 2 1 0	_____
4. Associates the use of the product with fun or pleasure.	5 4 3 2 1 0	_____
5. Associates the use of the product with being attractive.	5 4 3 2 1 0	_____
6. Encourages the use of the product as a method of problem-solving.	5 4 3 2 1 0	_____
7. Suggests that everyone is using the product.	5 4 3 2 1 0	_____
8. Suggests that people who use the product are mature.	5 4 3 2 1 0	_____
9. Shows a model using the product.	5 4 3 2 1 0	_____
10. Suggests that the product will improve performance (intellectual, physical, spiritual, etc.).	5 4 3 2 1 0	_____

Total Points _____

(continued...)

© ETR Associates

MEDIA MESSAGES

CONTINUED

SCORING AND INTERPRETATION OF RESULTS

Step 1. Add the points for each statement.

Step 2. After you have added up the total points, place an X on the following line at the spot that best represents the total points.

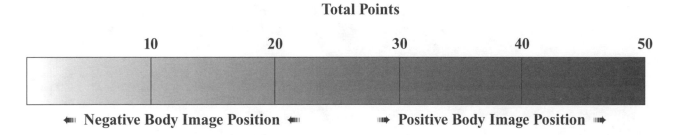

Total Points

Negative Body Image Position ◀◀◀   ▶▶▶ Positive Body Image Position ▶▶▶

Step 3. Comment on your analysis or evaluation of the body image messages in the advertisement.

© ETR Associates

CHECK YOUR KNOWLEDGE

Name _____ Date _____ Period _____

DIRECTIONS → Read each of the statements. Circle *T* if the statement is *completely* true. Circle *F* if the statement is completely or even partly false.

T F 1. Teens may develop unusual eating behaviors as a way to become independent and rebel against authority, such as parents and teachers.

T F 2. Eating a lot of food in a short time is called bingeing.

T F 3. Insisting that your body is fat, even when you're very thin, is a symptom of anorexia nervosa.

T F 4. Being teased by friends about being fat or needing to diet can trigger an eating disorder.

T F 5. Thinking about food all the time is a symptom of eating disorders.

T F 6. Feeling depressed often is a symptom of eating disorders.

T F 7. Losing too much weight due to starvation is a symptom of bulimia.

T F 8. Most weight-loss diets provide normal ways to eat for a lifetime.

T F 9. Forcing yourself to vomit is one of the common behaviors of bulimia.

T F 10. Only females are affected by eating disorders.

T F 11. Diet pills are a good way to help people lose weight and keep it off.

T F 12. People can become addicted to diet pills.

T F 13. People with eating disorders have low self-esteem.

T F 14. Most people with anorexia nervosa deny that their eating behavior is a serious problem.

T F 15. People with eating disorders believe that a thin body will bring them happiness and success.

© ETR Associates

Choosing Health High School

WHAT CAUSES EATING DISORDERS?

STUDENT READING

Many teenagers believe that dieting is the normal way to eat. Magazines, billboards, movies, television shows and commercials all seem to send the message that being thin leads to happiness, success, self-confidence and respect.

People with eating disorders believe these messages. They spend a lot of their time and energy thinking about what they eat and how they look. They focus so much on their appearance they often don't develop confidence and abilities in other areas.

PSYCHOLOGICAL FACTORS

People who have eating disorders have a negative body image. They tend to have low self-esteem and feel inadequate. They often work hard to prove they are good enough, because deep down they're afraid they aren't. They tend to be competitive and ambitious. They want to be perfect. They think that if they are thin, they will be happy, popular, successful and confident.

FAMILY PROBLEMS

Some teens use eating disorders as an excuse to remain dependent on their parents. They may be afraid to grow up and leave the safety of school and their families. Others use their unusual food behaviors as a way to assert their independence and rebel against family standards.

An eating disorder can be a way to protest against strict parents. In some families, the teen feels he or she has to take care of the parents, and does not want this unfair responsibility.

LIFESTYLE FACTORS

People with eating disorders tend to not be very assertive. They usually don't handle stress well. They often don't have goals (other than weight loss) that can help them feel independent and self-confident.

They may have friends who are also very concerned about physical appearance and thinness. Many dancers, actresses, models, gymnasts, flight attendants, sorority members and jockeys have eating disorders.

BIOLOGICAL FACTORS

There may be biological reasons some people are more likely to develop an eating disorder. These biological factors may be related to alcoholism or depression. People with certain types of eating disorders may abuse alcohol and other drugs.

There is an increased risk of eating disorders if a close relative has had one. Some families have a greater tendency toward obesity than others.

NUTRITION

Dieting or limiting eating over a long time can put body processes out of balance. Changes in the body can lead to eating disorders. But most physical problems are results, not causes, of eating disorders.

Poor nutrition causes changes in the way the body uses calories from food. These changes can make it harder to lose weight and easier to gain it. The frustration this causes can lead people to overeat (binge), then try to get rid of the food by purging. But this just makes the problem worse.

TRIGGERS

Many of the factors that contribute to eating disorders can exist for years before anything happens. But then something sets off a cycle of strict dieting or bingeing and purging. The event that sets off this cycle is called a *trigger*.

Trigger incidents are usually problems the person is not prepared to handle. Triggers can include losses, such as death, divorce or leaving home; school pressures; a long-distance move; or the break-up of an important relationship. Many teens with eating disorders report that teasing from their peers or comments about their bodies made them decide they were fat and needed to diet.

Many people with eating disorders are also victims of rape, incest, verbal abuse and neglect. They don't know how to express their fear, rage, confusion and need for help. So they turn to or away from food. They may use food for comfort. Or they may go on strict diets to help them feel in control of their lives.

© ETR Associates

What Is Anorexia Nervosa?

Student Reading

Anorexia nervosa is a serious eating disorder. People with this disorder say they feel fat or that parts of their body are fat, even if they weigh much less than is normal or healthy.

Some people are just naturally very thin. This doesn't mean they are anorexic. What sets people with anorexia nervosa apart are their attitudes about food and their desire to be even thinner. People with anorexia nervosa are very concerned about their body size and are usually unhappy with some feature of their physical appearance. They spend a lot of time thinking about eating, food, weight and body image.

They may count calories, weigh themselves many times a day and go on strict diets, even if they are very thin. They may feel uncomfortable after eating a normal or even a very small meal. They may think of foods as good or bad. They may also judge how well they control their eating habits and measure their success in terms of how much weight they can lose.

People with anorexia nervosa usually lose weight by fasting and/or reducing the amount of food they eat and exercising a lot. Some may make themselves vomit or use laxatives or diuretics to lose weight.

Other peculiar behaviors around food are also common. People with anorexia nervosa often fix special meals for others, but limit themselves to a few low-calorie foods. They may hide food or throw it away.

Some anorexics may feel compelled to wash their hands frequently or behave in other unusual ways. Most people with anorexia nervosa don't believe they have a problem with food.

The problem usually begins in the early to late teens and is often related to stress. It occurs most often in females. Only about one-third of them are slightly overweight before the problem begins. The disorder is more common among people who have sisters and mothers who are anorexic.

Many people have only one episode of anorexia nervosa and then return to normal eating patterns and weight. But in some cases, weight loss is so severe that the person has to be put in the hospital to prevent death by starvation; 5–18% of people with anorexia nervosa die from the disorder.

© ETR Associates

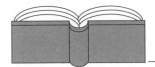

WHAT IS BULIMIA?

STUDENT READING

Bulimia is an eating disorder that involves bingeing and purging. Bingeing (binge eating) is eating a large amount of food in a short period of time. Purging refers to trying to get rid of the food that's been eaten by vomiting or using laxatives or diuretics.

People with bulimia often feel they are out of control during binges. They find it hard to resist the urge to binge or to stop once they've started. They also may try other ways to prevent weight gain, including strict diets, diet aids, fasts or lots of exercise.

Some people with bulimia may plan their eating binges. They buy sweet, high-calorie food to eat during the binge. This food may also be easy to eat quickly, without a lot of chewing, such as ice cream. The binge is usually kept hidden from others. Once the binge has begun, the person may look for more food to eat when the food that started the binge is gone.

A binge usually ends when the binger's stomach starts to hurt or if someone interrupts. After bingeing, many bulimics make themselves vomit to purge the food. Vomiting usually reduces the stomach pain. Then the person starts eating again or ends the binge. Sometimes the binge ends with the person going to sleep.

Some people with bulimia binge in order to vomit or vomit after eating only a small amount of food. Although a binge may seem enjoyable at the time, the person often feels depressed afterwards.

Binges usually alternate with times of normal eating. When the problem gets worse, the person may binge or fast with no periods of normal eating. A person who averages 2 or more binge-eating episodes a week for at least 3 months is considered bulimic.

The problem usually begins in adolescence or early adult life. People with bulimia are typically within a normal weight range. But whatever they weigh, they are very concerned about weight and body image. Their lives are dominated by conflicts around eating and their weight may change often due to the alternating binges and fasts. Although the long-term outcome of bulimia is not known, vomiting may harm the teeth, stomach and esophagus, and cause chemical imbalances and dehydration.

© ETR Associates

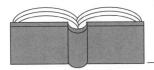

DRUGS AND EATING DISORDERS

STUDENT READING

People with eating disorders may abuse several types of drugs.

LAXATIVES

Laxatives seem to move food through the body more rapidly. They may relieve stomach bloating and pain after a binge. But they don't prevent the calories in food from being absorbed. Any weight loss is due mostly to loss of water and minerals and is only temporary.

Misuse of laxatives is harmful:

- They upset the body's mineral balance.
- They lead to dehydration (not enough water in the cells of the body).
- They damage the lining of the digestive tract.
- They let the digestive tract get lazy. Someone who uses laxatives regularly may become constipated without them.

DIURETICS

Diuretics, or water pills, help the body get rid of excess water by increasing the amount of urine. They can cause sudden weight loss. But they also cause dehydration. Diuretics are dangerous. They increase the loss of important minerals—calcium, potassium, magnesium and zinc—from the body. In a rebound effect, they can also cause the body to retain salt and water, and make it more sensitive to diet changes.

IPECAC SYRUP

Ipecac syrup is taken to cause vomiting. It has been linked to the deaths of several people with eating disorders. The active ingredient (emetine) can build up in body tissues and cause muscle or heart weakness. Ipecac is toxic (poisonous), whether taken in a large amount or small amounts that build up over time.

DIET PILLS

Pills are often taken to help with weight loss. The best known pills are Dexedrine and Benzedrine. These require a prescription from a doctor. But the FDA prohibits doctors from prescribing these drugs for weight loss.

Some over-the-counter drugs, available without a prescription, can also be used to temporarily reduce appetite. But usually the appetite returns to normal after a week or so, and the lost weight is gained back. Then the user has the problem of trying to get off the drug without gaining more weight.

Drugs do not really help people lose weight and keep it off. They can be addictive, and lead to dangerous physical problems if misused.

© ETR Associates

PRIVACY CIRCLES

Name _____ Date _____ Period _____

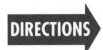 **DIRECTIONS** In the center circle, identify the person in whom you would be most likely to confide. Identify the second most likely person in the second circle, and so on. Then draw a line from each situation to the circle that shows the person with whom you would share that information.

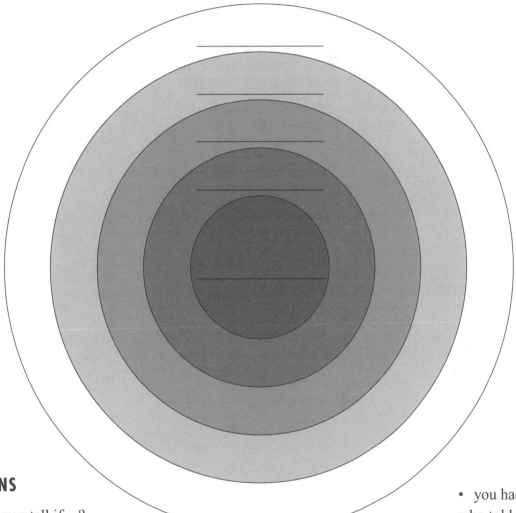

SITUATIONS

Who would you tell if…?

• you were in love

• you had a friend who vomited in the school restroom to control his or her weight

• your friend was stealing money from parents or friends to buy food to binge on

• you got a new job

• you had a friend who told you he or she was thinking about committing suicide

• you had a friend who was starving herself or himself to lose weight

© ETR Associates

- **Learn to like yourself, just as you are.**

- **Set realistic goals for yourself.**

- **Ask for support and encouragement from friends and family when life is stressful.**

- **Learn the basics of good nutrition and exercise.**

- **If you want to lose weight, talk to a doctor or a professional, registered dietitian who specializes in weight control.**

- **Seek adult help if you suspect you or a friend has an eating disorder problem.**

© ETR Associates

HELP FOR EATING DISORDERS

NATIONAL NONPROFIT EATING DISORDERS ORGANIZATIONS

AABA
American Anorexia/Bulimia Association
418 E. 76th Street
New York, NY 10021
(212) 734-1114

ABC
Anorexia Bulimia Care, Inc.
545 Concord Avenue
Cambridge, MA 02138-1122
(617) 492-7670

ANAD
National Association of Anorexia Nervosa and Associated Disorders
P.O. Box 7
Highland Park, IL 60035
(847) 831-3438

ANRED
Anorexia Nervosa and Related Eating Disorders
P.O. Box 5102
Eugene, OR 97405
(503) 344-1144

EDAP
Eating Disorders Awareness and Prevention
255 Alhambra Circle, #321
Coral Gables, FL 33134
(305) 444-3731

F.E.E.D.
Foundation for Education about Eating Disorders
5238 Duvall Drive
Bethesda, MD 20816

IAEDP
International Association of Eating Disorders Professionals
123 NW 13th Street, #206
Boca Raton, FL 33432-1618
(800) 800-8126

NAAS
National Anorexic Aid Society
1925 E. Dublin-Granville Road
Columbus, OH 43229
(614) 436-1112

OA
Overeaters Anonymous Headquarters
World Services Office
P.O. Box 92870
Los Angeles, CA 90009
(310) 618-8835

© ETR Associates

PROBLEMS EATING YOU?

Name _____ Date _____ Period _____

DIRECTIONS ➤ Read the following statements. Circle *Yes* if the statement describes someone you know. Circle *No* if it doesn't apply.

I have a friend who…

1. Constantly thinks about eating, weight and body size.	Yes	No
2. Feels anxious before eating.	Yes	No
3. Is terrified of being overweight.	Yes	No
4. Doesn't know when he or she is hungry.	Yes	No
5. Goes on eating binges and can't stop eating until she or he feels sick.	Yes	No
6. Says she or he feels bloated or uncomfortable after eating.	Yes	No
7. Spends a lot of time daydreaming about food.	Yes	No
8. Weighs herself or himself several times a day.	Yes	No
9. Exercises a lot and gets very uptight about his or her exercise plan.	Yes	No
10. Says that being in control of food shows self-control.	Yes	No
11. Has taken laxatives or forced herself or himself to vomit after eating.	Yes	No
12. Is letting food control his or her life.	Yes	No
13. Says she or he feels very guilty after eating.	Yes	No
14. Eats when feeling nervous, anxious, lonely or depressed.	Yes	No
15. Doesn't think he or she looks good in clothes.	Yes	No
16. Seems uptight about her or his weight and appearance when around other people.	Yes	No
17. Seems resentful when a friend or family member talks about her or his eating habits.	Yes	No
18. Tries to diet for a definite period of time, but never seems to make it all the way.	Yes	No
19. Avoids parties and get-togethers because of feeling self-conscious about weight.	Yes	No
20. Has a problem with overeating and doesn't know what to do.	Yes	No

© ETR Associates

JEOPARDY GAME BOARD

POINTS	TERMS (Unit 1)	CULTURE AND MEDIA (Unit 2)	EATING DISORDERS (Unit 3)	HELP FOR EATING DISORDERS (Unit 4)	POTPOURRI (All Units)
10	The way you view and believe others view your body	Means of communication that convey messages to the public	Disorder characterized by self-imposed starvation and refusal to maintain or gain weight	A course of action to stop a disease	Ability to critically interpret messages from the media
20	A measure of how you value yourself	10% or more above desirable weight	Absence or cessation of menstruation	Conforming with an accepted standard; natural	An event that sets off a cycle of strict dieting or bingeing and purging
30	Traits, including physical, mental/emotional, social and personality traits	Ideas, customs, skills and arts of a people or group	Disorder characterized by binge eating followed by purging, fasting or exercise	Anything that triggers a stress response	An image or model thought of as perfect
40	Psychological well-being; the capacity to cope with life situations	Condition in which an excessive proportion of body tissue is fat; 20% or more above desirable weight	Eating a very large amount of food at one time	Sharing sensitive or personal information with another person	Members give emotional help, share experience, exchange information; used in addition to primary treatment
50	Characteristics that provide a sense of self and others	★Double Points★ Media; family and cultural perceptions; physical characteristics; and self-esteem ★Double Points★	Attempts to rid body of food (vomiting, laxative, and/or diuretic abuse)	Like yourself as you are. Set realistic goals. Learn about nutrition and exercise. Ask for support. Seek help.	★Double Points★ 4 drugs abused by people with eating disorders ★Double Points★

© ETR Associates

Choosing Health High School